AgeLess

Living Younger Longer

AgeLess

Living Younger Longer

BEN H. DOUGLAS

QRP BOOKS
Brandon, Mississippi

Library of Congress Cataloging-in-Publication Data

Douglas, Ben H.
   AgeLess / by Ben H. Douglas.
      p. cm.
   ISBN 0-937552-33-x : $12.95
   1. Longevity. 2. Aging. 3. Health. I. Title. II. Title:
AgeLess.
   QP85.D68 1990
   612.6'7--dc20   89-70325
                                                        CIP

Quail Ridge Press / QRP Books
P.O. Box 123
Brandon, MS 39043

To Ben and Nell Douglas
for being good parents to Paul, Ellen, and me.

Contents

Acknowledgments

A number of very capable people contributed to this project. I am grateful to all of them. Mrs. Peggy Maclain tracked down references in the medical literature, provided essential secretarial assistance, and remained organized through it all.

The editors and publishers at QRP Books could not have done a finer job. Gwen and Barney McKee insisted that we strive for perfection, kept the overall project in perspective, and kept us clearly on course. The personnel at QRP Books have become more than business associates. . .they have become friends.

My special thanks to the many members of the faculty and staff of the University of Mississippi Medical Center who so generously helped and encouraged me.

Final thanks go to Alice for her support, and to my friends and family for their support and encouragement.

Preface

You can determine, to a great extent, the rate at which you age. I confess that this came as quite a surprise to me when I first began to see the evidence for it. I, like so many others, believed that the aging process was completely beyond our control.

A multitude of things which are blamed on the aging process have nothing whatsoever to do with aging. They are a result of abuse and disuse. This book makes a clear distinction between the changes caused by aging and the ones which are caused by neglect.

Myths about aging abound. As you study through this material, you will see many myths dispelled. You will see why some people are young at the age of 70 and others are old at the age of 50. You will find that you can choose to be young or old at any given chronological age. You will see why, in the future, it's going to be commonplace for 70-year olds to put on their jeans, jump into their sports cars and go to the gym for a workout. Other things will become apparent.

You will find that delaying the aging process stretches out the "middle years" of life, that older individuals are not all alike, that aging is partly a matter of choice, and that aging may be partly psychosomatic. You will learn how to avoid chronic fatigue and have a super-charged body. You will find that intense mental activity and a power of purpose can affect the rate at which you age. You will learn about the effects of *proper* diet and exercise on the body.

Ways to prevent the premature aging of every single system of your body will be explored. Some exciting research that has allowed scientists to slow the aging clocks of experimental animals will be described.

The information presented has been documented by scientific research or clinical trials. On the rare occasion when I speculate about something, it is clearly labeled as speculation.

Can we slow the aging clock now? Yes. Legitimate scientists don't claim that they can make people live forever. They do know that it's possible to intervene and prevent and/or inhibit many of the processes associated with aging.

Read this book and take charge of your life. Stay young right to the very end of your life span.

Ben H. Douglas

About the Author

Dr. Ben Douglas is currently professor of anatomy, professor of obstetrics and gynecology (research), and director of the graduate program at the University of Mississippi Medical Center in Jackson. He received his doctorate in physiology and biophysics from that institution and was appointed to the medical faculty in 1964. He has been actively involved in teaching, research, and administration since that time.

He has published more than 250 journal articles, book chapters and abstracts of his presentations. His scientific articles have appeared in 28 different medical journals, including the *American Journal of Physiology,* the *American Journal of Obstetrics and Gynecology,* and *Endocrinology.* His particular research interest is the effect of the dietary intake of minerals and nutrients on blood pressure, body weight and atherosclerosis.

Dr. Douglas is currently the President of the Society for the Study of Pathophysiology of Pregnancy, an international organization consisting of 4,500 scientists from 70 countries. He is a member of eleven professional societies, including the Society for Gynecologic Investigation, the American Physiological Society and the American Federation for Clinical Research. He has served as a review editor for several medical journals and is currently on the editorial board of *Clinical and Experimental Hypertension.*

Dr. Douglas has presented the results for his research before such diverse groups as the Polish Gynecological Society (Szczecin, Poland, 1980), the Society of Pathophysiology of Pregnancy (Dubrovnik, Yugoslavia, 1980), and the Japanese Hypertension Society (Sendai, Japan, 1985.) He has researched, written and delivered more than 100 scientific lectures to medical groups throughout the United States and to medical groups in Germany, Israel, Switzerland, Austria, the Netherlands, Ireland, Scotland, Italy, and Egypt.

Because of the significant data which Dr. Douglas' research has generated, he has received a number of honors and awards. Early in his career, he served for a year as a Visiting Investigator at the Medical Research Council Blood Pressure Unit at the Western Infirmary in Glasgow, Scotland. In 1972 he was named an Established Investigator of the American Heart Association. In 1978 he received the American Heart Association-Mississippi Affiliate Silver Distinguished Achievement Award. In 1983 he received the Mississippi Academy of Sciences Award for Outstanding Contribution to Science. He served that organization as president in 1985.

Dr. Douglas is the author of the very popular weight control book, *Reset Your Appestat*. He has also authored two medical books and is a contributing author to four others.

Introduction

A 1O-POINT SYSTEM FOR STAYING YOUNG

Inhibiting the aging process is a do-it-yourself project. When you undertake any project, you naturally want to be able to periodically determine what progress you are making toward your goal. The goal in this case is *to be as young and healthy as possible, whatever your age.* When you use the scoring system which is outlined below, it will be relatively easy for you to see how well you are doing. The scoring system is based on the "perfect 10" concept. It has become fairly common in our society to rate a number of things—athletic events and human attractiveness, included—on the basis of 10. Ten is perfect. Anything less is. . .well, you get the idea.

When it comes to inhibiting the aging process, there are certain things that we can do *for* ourselves and there are things that we can do *to* ourselves. When we do good things for ourselves, we add points to our score. If we do harmful things to ourselves, we subtract points. It's that simple.

At this point I want to tell you about the scoring system. (This book describes in detail what is meant by adequate aerobic exercise, a good diet, stimulating the brain and the other things listed.) You can be as relaxed or as precise about the scoring as you wish.

When you close your eyes at night, you can mentally think, "I ate right, exercised, didn't have too much alcohol, etc. I treated my body right. I give myself a 9." It will be easy and automatic. Or you can be more precise. You can get a calendar with squares and fill in a score each day. Then you can calculate your average score for a week, month or year. Either method will allow you to determine how you are doing toward inhibiting your aging process.

Use the following chart to determine how well you are doing at inhibiting the aging process which is taking place in your body:

INHIBITING AGING

PLUS (points)		MINUS (points)	
Maintain good diet	+3	Consume excessive	
Get aerobic exercise.	+2	fatty foods.	-2
Stimulate brain.	+2	Drink excess alcohol. .	-2
Break mental barriers		Smoke.	-2
and dispel myths	+1	Getting stressed.	-1
Get adequate water intake. .	+1	Too much sun.	-1
Get adequate rest	+1	Irregular meals and	
		junk foods.	-1
		Inattention to health	
		care needs.	-1
TOTAL	+10	TOTAL	-10

You can see how the scoring system works. If on a given day you do everything listed in the left column, your score would be +10, *unless* you also did some of the things listed in the column on the right. For example if you earn a +10 but you smoke and have too much alcohol, that drops your score to +6.

Certain other things become apparent. If you smoke you can never get above a +8. If you eat junk food on the run every day, you can never get above a +9. These scores will give you a good idea of how well you are personally inhibiting your own aging process.

WHERE YOU STAND

SCORE		COMMENTS
9 - 10	Ideal.	You are inhibiting the aging process.
7 - 8	Good.	You are a health-conscious person.
5 - 6	Fair.	There is definite room for improvement.
0 - 4	Poor.	Your body needs help.
-1 to -10		Keep paying your life insurance premiums.

Now as you read on you will learn what the aging process is all about. You will learn how to do the things that will give you plus points.

AgeLess

Living Younger Longer

CHAPTER 1

Breaking Barriers
and Dispelling Myths

Some time ago I saw a humorous anecdote in the newspaper about a 94-year-old man who was visiting his physician. The physician, after confirming that his patient was in good general health, proceeded to list the bad health practices that the man was following. Finally, the patient conceded and said to the doctor, "Doc, if I had known I was going to live this long, I would've taken better care of myself."

Often our bodies are capable of doing remarkable things in spite of the way we treat them. Imagine what they could do if they had our full, enthusiastic support and attention.

The body that you have is the vehicle that is going to carry you through life. It will be with you every second of your journey on this planet. Maybe there are some things about your body that you would change. Perhaps you think it is too large, or too small, or too young (a thought that only a *very* young person would have), or too old. Whatever you might think of your body, it's yours. You can't *exchange* your body for another, but, if you wish, you can *change* the one that you have. The accomplished comedian Flip Wilson, when playing the part of the siren Geraldine, frequently quips, "What you see is what you get!" Well, sometimes what you see *is* what you get.

How do you see your body?

Do you see it as one that can't change? Do you see it as an oversized, tired old smoking piece of machinery that is so clogged and sluggish it can barely get you from one place to another? Do you see it as one which will soon wear out and be consigned to the junk heap? Or do you see your body as a finely tuned instrument that is physically and mentally fit; and has abundant energy; that has a constant intake of high-quality nutrients to keep its engines purring and performing at peak efficiency; and that is going to last for a long time to come? If your body isn't a finely tuned machine now, you can begin to turn it into one *today.*

If your body *is* an oversized, tired old piece of machinery that is clogged and sluggish, do you want to change it? Do you want to again have that vitality that gives you the feeling you can take on the world? You can have that feeling. Do you remember how it felt when, after a hard-fought, energy-draining game, you walked off the court or off the athletic field still feeling terrific and full of life? Would you like to feel that way again? You can. Or, if you are one of those fortunate individuals whose body is now fit and full of energy, do you want to keep it that way for a longer time than you ever thought possible? You can. The level of fitness and energy that you can achieve will surprise you.

How can we realize our full potential?

We are just beginning to realize our potential for extended, productive, creative living. We learn about the human body and its life span by using the scientific laboratory, by studying different cultures and by observing individuals who have themselves led full and exciting lives.

From the scientific laboratory information comes daily regarding chemical reactions responsible for the life processes in the cells of the human body. The intricate mechanisms which control the entire life process of the cells are being carefully studied.

Humans begin life as one-celled organisms. That cell divides into two cells, then into four, and so on. Finally some of the cells change to liver cells, some to muscle cells, and others to the various types of cells found in the body. These changes have been intensively studied by research scientists. There is little doubt that the entire process is carefully programmed. This highly complex program makes it possible for some cell types to grow, multiply, and change, while other cell types disappear when they are no longer needed. The process is nothing short of miraculous. It is a programmed change. The blueprint for the process is built into the genes.

Is aging a programmed event?

When humans reach maturity, the programmed changes in the life process continue. Both the developmental period and the aging process following maturity are probably programmed in a similar fashion. If aging occurred just because the programmed maturity phase stopped, then all animals would age at approximately the same rate. They don't. The conclusion is inescapable: aging, like maturation, is a programmed event. The more we can learn about the "aging clock"—about how maturation and aging are regulated—the more likely the possibility that we can use that information to our advantage to slow the aging clock and increase our life span. The daily accumulation of knowledge from the research laboratory brings us closer and closer to that possibility.

What about superlongevity?

We are learning more about longevity and extended productivity by studying different cultures. Even acknowledging the fact that there are myths about superlongevity (people who live to be 130, 140 or even 160 years old), it is a fact that there are population groups in the world with a disproportionate number of centenarians.

The Andean villages in Ecuador are said to have a high proportion of centenarians, and there are also widely publicized accounts of individuals who live to a very old age in the Soviet Caucasus Mountains and in the Altai Mountains in Siberia. There have been reports of superlongevity from Brazil, Pakistan, Kenya, and the Nepalese mountains. The birth records of these individuals who claim to be 130 or more years old are questionable, but there are geographical areas where a higher percentage of the people have a longer life expectancy than in most other parts of the world. The current official world record of longevity, which is considered valid in some scientific journals, belongs to a Japanese, Shigechio Izumi of Kyushu, who died at the age of 119 in 1984. (The unofficial record, which many Soviet scientific publications consider valid, belongs to Shiralibaba Muslimov, who lived in the Caucasus. His death at the age of 168 was reported in many newspapers around the world.) When Florence Knapp of Lansdale, Pennsylvania, reached the age of 113, she was said to be the oldest living person in the United States. The records aside, there are more than 25,000 centenarians in the United States. We can learn much from them. We have learned how and why people can be alert and active even though they have reached the age of 100.

Why look at individuals?

We can also learn by observing individuals. At the 44th Annual Meeting of the American Geriatrics Society, Ida Kohlmeyer, a nationally recognized artist, said, "With maturity comes belief in yourself and the courage to take chances and to make changes in your style." (So much for the thought that only the young have the vigor and adventuresome spirit to take chances.) Individuals who attended that same meeting learned a lesson in "looking forward" from Danny Barker, a jazz musician who has performed with Louis Armstrong, Jelly Roll Morton, and the De Paris Brothers. Danny said, "Jazz keeps me alive. When I've got a gig, the pains leave; my whole attitude changes."

So it is with most of us. When we are looking forward to something, our pains leave and we become more alive.

We learn about the possibilities of extended physical activity from individuals such as John Boots, who began competitive running at age 63 and now holds a number of U.S. and world records. His recommendation: "Be as physically active as you can within your health limits, and don't be afraid to take up something new in your later years." Perhaps the age of 63 seems a bit late in life to begin some new type of physical activity, but is it? Not really, when you consider that the age of 63 is only just past the midway point of the human life span.

Florence Knapp, at the age of 113 said, "There's nothing wrong with me. I might make it to 200."

What is aging anyway?

According to Webster's, to age is "to become old; to show the effects or the characteristics of increasing age." If we use that definition of aging, we can see that some people "age" and others, for all practical purposes, refuse to do so. Luck has very little to do with it. Those people who don't age, do things differently from those people who do age. The average person probably takes advantage of about 10 percent of the known factors that can lead to a longer, healthier, more productive life. By taking advantage of 100 percent of those factors, the same individuals could undergo an astonishing physical and mental transformation.

That is the message of this book: *increase the all-out effort to obtain the maximum advantage for your body from 10 percent to 100 percent and thereby insure for yourself a longer, healthier, more active life.* This will involve nothing mystical. It will involve breaking some mental and physical barriers (which we will find aren't barriers after all), taking advantage of the new information on nutrition, appreciating the importance of continued intense mental activity, taking a new approach to physical activity, eliminating undesirable stress, and utilizing the new information gained from the latest medical research.

A key ingredient in making this transition is to believe that you *can* do the things required to dramatically inhibit any premature aging which may be taking place in your body right now. The importance of a high degree of confidence cannot be overstated. There is very little difference between what we *believe* we can do and what we actually *can* do. That is especially true in this situation.

What is the first step toward preventing premature aging?

Before we can begin to prevent premature aging, it is essential that we break through a mental barrier that has plagued us for so long. *We must abolish the myth that we will become "old" when we have reached a certain chronological age.*

How old is old?

Years ago, people were considered to be old when they reached their 50s. It became a self-fulfilling prophecy. When they reached that age they took it easy. As a result, joints stiffened, muscles weakened, metabolism slowed, and other signs of aging appeared. Then the term "old age" applied to the mid- to late 60s. People waited until then to take it easy and get old. They put off having stiffened joints, weakened muscles, and slowed metabolism for a period of 10 to 15 years. It seems that if the population can postpone the aging process once, it can do so again. That is why I want to emphasize the importance of breaking this mental barrier and urge you to be optimistic that you can do it. Let me explain this a bit further.

Optimism, according to Webster's is ". . .an inclination to put the most favorable construction upon actions and events or to *anticipate the best possible outcome."* Since there is very little difference between what we believe we can do and what we can do, anticipating a particular outcome will make that outcome more probable.

Can optimism help prevent premature aging?

The balance between optimism and pessimism has a lot to do with one's ability to tolerate frustration, stress, and depression, all of which may bring on premature aging. As long as a person doesn't have unreasonable expectations ("If I jump out the window, I am sure I can fly") and takes reasonable precautions ("I'd better not drive fast on this wet street"), expecting the best possible outcome of a situation can usually influence that outcome. There are some physiological reasons for this which will be discussed in more detail later, one of which is worth mentioning here: positive, exciting mental images and expectations are associated with elevated blood levels of endorphins, and those endorphins make it easier to cope with frustrating, stressful situations.

Let us begin the process of breaking down some barriers. Gerontologists recognize the importance of accepting the idea that *aging is partly a matter of choice.* Speaking before a meeting of the American Academy of Family Physicians, Dr. Alex Comfort, author and gerontologist, argued that 75 percent of so-called aging results from a kind of self-fulfilling prophecy (quoted from: Conniff, R., in *Aging*, p. 49, 4th Edition, H. Cox, Editor, Dushkin Publishing Co., Guilford, CT). Dr. Comfort said, "If we insist that there is a group of people who, on a fixed calendar basis, cease to be people and become unintelligent, asexual, unemployable, and crazy, the people so designated will be under pressure to *be* unintelligent, asexual, unemployable, and crazy."

Is aging partly psychosomatic?

Lawrence Casler, a psychologist from State University College in Geneseo, New York is so convinced that aging is psychosomatic that he gave a powerful hypnotic suggestion to 150 young volunteers that they would live to at least 120. He did this so they could break through the "brainwashing" about life span. They are planning a party for the year 2070. Casler went a step further. He gave a hypnotic suggestion for long life to residents of a nursing home who were more than 80 years of age. A similar group received no hypnotherapy and served as the control group. The group which received the hypnotic suggestion lived an average of two years longer than the control group. (Conniff, p.49).

On the very day that I was writing about barriers, I had the opportunity to talk to Sir Roger Bannister, the first person ever to run the mile in less than four minutes. He is now Master of Pembroke College in Oxford, England, and is Consultant Physician at the National Hospital for Nervous Diseases in London. I spoke to him when he came to the University of Mississippi Medical Center to give some lectures on diseases of the nervous system.

Before Sir Roger ran the sub-four-minute mile, it was considered by athletes and nonathletes alike as a barrier that was beyond the limits of human endurance. Apparently, young Roger Bannister was concentrating on his race with such intensity that he didn't think about the "barrier," and so did what had been previously considered impossible. Since that time, the feat has been repeated hundreds of times. Just as Roger Bannister did away with a barrier, perhaps we can do away with another "barrier"—the belief that humans *must* become "old" at a certain chronological age.

Can I age more slowly than the average person?

One problem with breaking through the aging barrier is that we are constantly bombarded with information about what the average person does as he ages. We are told that the average person's body weight is going to increase by 8 to 10 percent; that when he is in his early 20s his body will be 15 percent fat, and that as he approaches 70 his body will be 30 percent fat; that the trim waist he has at the age of 20 will expand by an average of six inches by the time he reaches 70; that because his heart, lungs, and muscles don't perform as well as they once did, his stamina will decrease by an average of 30 to 40 percent by the age of 70; and that his height will decrease by approximately 1.6 percent (about one and one-fourth inches for a man who is six feet tall) by the time he reaches the age of 70.

Fine. Let the average person do what he will. Recent developments clearly demonstrate that *you can practice to avoid being average.* You not only can rewrite the statistics concerning what the average person does as he gets older, you can practice to do things that you aren't supposed to be able to do. Your body weight doesn't have to increase, the percent of your body weight that is fat doesn't have to increase, your trim waistline doesn't have to get larger, and your stamina doesn't have to decrease 30 to 40 percent.

Even the statistics for the decrease in height are not chiseled in stone. That information was obtained by examining 70-year-olds who during their midlife, were admonished to "take it easy" so as not to place undue physical stress on their bodies. They usually complied because they were responding to the medical opinion which prevailed at the time. The proper balance of "good" stress in the form of physical activity, plus the continually improving nutrition of individuals, will probably significantly alter the data on changes in height with age.

How exactly does the "average" person age?

We are told that the reflexes of the average person decrease by approximately 8 percent between the ages of 20 and 70; that his muscle strength decreases by 25 percent by the age of 70; that he loses 8 to 10 teeth by the age of 70. The muscles of respiration weaken and the joints of the chest cavity become less flexible in the average person as he gets older. These data raise the following questions: how much of the decrease in reflexes is a result of a lack of practice to keep the reflexes sharp? Would there be a decrease in muscle strength if the individuals had not been advised to "take it easy" during midlife? Modern dental science being what it is, is it not now possible for an individual to keep all of his teeth all of his life? Would the muscles of respiration weaken and the joints of the chest cavity become less flexible if they were exercised daily?

We are told that nerve cells are lost from the brain as a person gets older and that the average person takes longer to process information and make decisions; that there is a slight loss of memory; and that there might actually be a decline in intelligence quotient (IQ). But how much of that decrease in the brain activity occurs because the person doesn't get as much mental exercise as he once did? In the "power" IQ tests— tests where the questions are more difficult but an unlimited time is allowed to answer them—older individuals perform as well as, and often better than, younger individuals.

The human brain has billions of neurons, and many agree with Albert Einstein's estimate that the average person uses only about 10 percent of the neurons he has for creative endeavors. There is evidence that mental prowess can last well into an advanced age. That has been demonstrated time and again by individuals such as Frank Lloyd Wright, the architect who completed New York's Guggenheim Museum at the age of 89 and continued teaching until his death; by the classical guitarist, Andres Segovia, who did a world tour at the age of 93; and by Sir Robert Mayer, who at the age of 101 was still arranging concerts, and who stated emphatically that he intended to die in harness.

One of the largest barriers that we need to break through with respect to premature aging is the belief that heart and blood vessel (cardiovascular) disease is inevitable. Unfortunately, we have come to believe that cardiovascular disease is natural and common, and that it will be with us forever. Later in this book, a careful step-by-step, detailed proposal will be offered for eliminating cardiovascular disease. For now, let us spend a little time dispensing with the myth that it is a part of the natural process of living.

Does the heart "wear out" with age?

The heart of the average person supposedly gets weaker with age. The resting heart rate remains about the same as a person gets older, but the heart pumps 25 to 30 percent less blood each minute by the time the average person reaches the age of 70. When he exercises, his maximum heart rate is 25 percent less than it was when he was 20 years old.

Approximately two million people die each year in the United States, and almost half of those deaths are from cardiovascular diseases. For years we accepted that as an "inevitable consequence of aging." We are just becoming awakened to the fact that much cardiovascular disease is preventable.

We become alarmed, as we should, when we read that approximately 50,000 people die each year in automobile accidents. But while that is happening, approximately 20,000 people die *each week* of cardiovascular disease. There would be a tremendous public outcry if 20,000 people were dying each week from diseases such as acquired immune deficiency syndrome (AIDS), rheumatic fever, polio, or some exotic new disease process.

The extent to which we are willing to accept death by heart and blood vessel disease as inevitable can be seen in newspaper accounts of celebrities who die of heart disease in their 40s, 50s, or 60s. The accounts frequently report that the individuals have died of "natural" causes.

Heart disease is not natural, it is not inevitable, and it does not afford a merciful way to end one's life. Heart disease is a preventable national tragedy. It's incredible that the death of 20,000 people each week in the United States is not news.

People in their 30s and 40s die of heart and blood vessel disease, but many think of heart disease as a disease of the elderly. Perhaps the reason it is sometimes thought of as a disease of the elderly is that, even though the arteries begin to be clogged during the teen years, there are no symptoms. The rate at which the arteries become clogged is largely dependent upon what we do on a day-by-day basis. In fact, there may never be symptoms. Nearly 500,000 people die each year of heart and blood vessel disease without warning, without any previous indication that they have the disease.

The causes of most heart and blood vessel diseases are known, and the diseases are preventable. Most of the diseases can be attributed to the fact that we lead the "good life" here in the United States. If you have been living on conventional American diets since childhood, you can expect that the atherosclerotic process (hardening of the arteries) is taking place in your blood vessels right now. If you smoke and/or have high blood pressure, the process is taking place at an even faster rate.

What does diet have to do with cardiovascular disease?

We have come to believe that it is our "right" to eat "good" American food. People say things like, "I have to have something that will stick to my ribs for breakfast. I have to have my bacon and eggs. I have to have something solid for lunch, like a couple of hamburgers. Give me a big steak for dinner. Don't put any of that sissy food in front of me." While we do have the right to choose our food, we also have the right to decide whether or not we want to join the 20,000 people a week who succumb to heart and blood vessel disease.

We don't have to believe that the American way involves having heart disease, obesity, high blood pressure, and atherosclerosis. It's ironic that our nutritional problems arise because of too much of the wrong type of food, while the nutritional problems of the poorer countries in the world result from a scarcity of food.

People frequently say to me that great-uncle or grandmother or some other person was born in 1900 and didn't do all of the things that doctors and scientists are advocating today but is still alive and kicking. I am glad that their relative or acquaintance is alive and well, but the fact is that *59 percent of the people who were born in 1900 didn't live to the age of 65.*

Isn't cardiovascular disease inherited?

Another notion we need to dispel is that cardiovascular disease is inherited and "if you are going to get it, you are going to get it and there's nothing you can do about it."

Nothing could be further from the truth. The fact that a person has grandparents, aunts, uncles, or cousins who die of heart and blood vessel disease isn't proof in itself that heart disease is inherited. Obviously, if half of the people in the United States die of cardiovascular disease, every family of any size is going to be affected. If members of a family have been affected for several generations, it is easy to conclude that cardiovascular disease is "inherited."

There is a lot of evidence that this is not so. For example, when Eskimos who lived in Greenland moved to Denmark and changed their dietary habits, the incidence of cardiovascular disease in their families increased. When Japanese move to the United States and begin eating the typical American diet, the same thing happens. If heart disease were truly an inherited disease, then the incidence would not change when people move from one country to another. They would carry the inherited protection, or susceptibility, with them.

(There is an inherited disease, affecting approximately one in 500 people, that causes blood cholesterol to be high. It appears that medical treatment can now lower the blood cholesterol levels in these individuals.)

Maybe you and I already have some cardiovascular disease. We haven't always known how to avoid it. Since we now know what contributes to it, we can take steps to prevent its progression. What I am proposing at this point is that we completely do away with the myth that heart disease is inevitable.

Isn't stress a major cause of cardiovascular disease?

One other idea that we need to eliminate regarding cardiovascular disease is that if we eliminate stress, we can do whatever else we please and not worry about heart disease. Human beings were designed to adapt to stress. When properly used, stress can actually make us stronger.

If we exercise our muscles (stress them), then give them time to recover, they become stronger. That is a response natural to all animals. *Undue, prolonged, unnecessary* stress can cause permanent damage to the body, and this is the type of stress that we want to eliminate. In the meantime, let us not blame stress for all of our heart and blood vessel disease problems.

In his book, *Type A Behavior And Your Heart,* Dr. Myer Friedman tells of competitive, hard-driving, easily frustrated individuals (Type A) who are continually pressing to get to the top, and who are more susceptible to heart and blood vessel disease than their more relaxed counterparts. Undue stress might contribute to cardiovascular problems, but it is not the only cause. For example, executives have no more hypertension than blue collar workers of the same age. Also, a study of more than 1,500 men for a period of seven years showed that those with a Type A personality had no more heart attacks than those with a Type B (easy-going) personality (New England Journal of Medicine 304:65-70, 1981). Other studies which included larger groups of individuals within the same corporation have shown the same results. So we musn't think that it really isn't necessary to pay attention to some of the other changes in lifestyle as long as stress is controlled. It is an important factor but not the only one. Preventing heart disease is a bit more complicated than that.

Does everybody who "gets old" become senile?

Now that we have eliminated the cardiovascular disease barrier, let us dispel some myths so that we may prepare ourselves mentally to slow down the aging process. It is a myth that all people will become senile as they get older. All individuals *don't* become confused, disoriented, and forgetful with advancing age—at any rate not any more so than some people who are younger. If a younger person is anxious, we call it anxiety; if a younger person is depressed, we call it depression; and if a younger person is grief-stricken or is over-medicated on a drug which makes him tranquil and lethargic, we say that he is grief-stricken or that he is tranquil and lethargic. It is unfortunate that we tend to use the term "senility" when the same things happen to an older person. (It is true that atherosclerosis can progress to the point that, because of an insufficient oxygen supply to the brain, some of the brain cells die.

When that happens, the resultant behavioral changes are due to a blood vessel disease and *not* to automatic age-induced senility.) Lifestyle changes, particularly dietary ones, can go a long way toward eliminating "senility" which is caused by blood vessel disease.

There are literally tens of thousands of individuals who not only do not become senile as they get older but are dazzling examples of productivity.

Am I going to become forgetful, helpless, and inactive?

For some unexplained reason, we have been led to believe that as individuals get older, they will become forgetful, helpless, and inactive. Voluminous data and numerous personal examples show otherwise. One such example was Konrad Adenauer. Adenauer was born in Cologne, Germany. He studied law and was active in politics. Imprisoned by the Nazis when he was in his 60s, he later became, at the age of 73, the first chancellor of the Federal Republic of Germany. He held that post for 14 years; before resigning he helped West Germany achieve full independence, guided their economic recovery (which is still referred to as the "Economic Miracle"), and helped bring about the "Reconciliation Treaty" with France. Konrad Adenauer was not forgetful, helpless, or inactive.

We are also told that people become more apathetic as they get older. Apparently Mother Teresa, the Nobel Prize-winning missionary, never got that instruction. She was born in 1910 and, far from being apathetic, said that humans will be judged not on "how much we have done, but how much love we have put into our actions." As to the millions of other older people, the myth that they become apathetic as they get older can be quickly dispelled by a few visits to museums, art galleries, theaters, libraries, sporting events, political rallies, vacation resorts, concerts, social events, and religious services. Many people become *less* apathetic as they get older. They become more concerned and curious about the world around them.

Will age slow down my productivity?

Another misconception is that older people become nonproductive. You know people in your city and state who remain enormously productive as they get older. Among them are farmers, teachers, construction workers, attorneys, entertainers, physicians, artists, scientists, and businessmen and women. When we speak of continued productivity with advancing age, we typically use such examples as Dr. John Rock who at the age of 70, introduced "the Pill," and spent the next 20 years promoting it. Yet, there are millions of less well known, productive people in every area of human endeavor who, as they get older, continue to help keep the wheels of civilization turning.

Are all older people alike?

We have been led to believe that as people get older their minds wander, they can't learn anything new, they become feeble, and they go about their daily routine in a semistupor. We have been led to believe that they are inflexible, that they are all pretty much alike and that they all progress to the point that they sit around in a nursing home waiting to die.

Most people who get older do not end up in nursing homes. In fact, 95 percent of the people over the age of 65 are active members of society. As to the myth that they are all alike, the very opposite is the case. As individuals get older, they tend to "fan out." Their interests, hobbies, and occupations diverge. (If you want to see a group of people who are alike—a group that tends to walk, talk, act, think, and dress alike—make a quick visit to your local high school.)

Can I continue to learn in later life?

I. F. Stone, who was born in 1910, said, "There are great joys in one's later years—as many as there are in one's youth. One of them is *learning and studying.* The things you study have much more significance; you understand them more fully. I'm studying ancient Greek language and civilization. It's difficult work, but very rewarding." (Quoted from Conniff. See references. Italics mine.) After Stone learned ancient Greek, he was able to read in the original the basic sources for his book, *The Trial Of Socrates.*

You might think that the individuals I have mentioned are exceptions, that I am only presenting anecdotal evidence. The truth is that the individuals mentioned are exceptions only to the extent that they are well known. There are millions of other, older individuals who are not so well known, but who also are active, productive members of society.

Again, 95 percent of older individuals *are* active members of society.

So there you have it. You are not automatically going to become forgetful, helpless, apathetic, nonproductive, inactive, semistuporous, inflexible, and feeble. You need not reach the point where you will be unable to learn anything new, and you need not look forward only to sitting around in a nursing home waiting to die. It is important to reject the notion that at a particular age, you *must* exhibit characteristic physical signs and certain behavioral patterns. Forget about how the average older person has been described. You can write your own ticket.

Now, do you want to put the aging process "on hold"? Do you want your skin, muscles, bones, digestive, urinary, reproductive, cardiovascular, and nervous systems to stay younger longer than they otherwise would have, had they not received the proper care and attention from you? Do you want to look younger than your chronological age? Do you want to have more energy and experience less fatigue than other people your age? Do you want to be more alert and more inquisitive about your surroundings than the "average" person your age? Do you want to reduce your chances of getting heart disease and degenerative diseases as you get older? Good. Read on.

In researching the material for this book, I encountered some very exciting information. I want to share that information with you (and quote the sources so that you will be able to explore some areas in more detail if you wish.) After doing the research, I reached the following conclusions and am confident that you will too: (1) humans are designed to be young and vigorous to the very end of their life span, (2) it is now possible to increase life expectancy, and (3) it might be possible to lengthen the human life span beyond its current limit of approximately 110 years. Read and reread—daily if necessary—the following summary until you have it completely internalized. Doing that one thing alone will change forever the way you view the passing of your own years, will make you feel that you have more control over what happens to you, and will likely give you a good start on preventing the premature aging of your own body.

Summary

1. *It is a myth that I must be old at a certain chronological age.*

2. *Let the average person do what he will; I refuse to be average when it comes to aging.*

3. *It is a myth that cardiovascular disease is inherited or inevitable.*

4. *It is a myth that all people become senile as they get older.*

5. *It is a myth that I will become forgetful, helpless, and inactive as I get older.*

6. *It is a myth that I will become apathetic, nonproductive, semi-stuporous, inflexible, and feeble as I get older.*

7. *Older people are not all alike.*

8. *Aging is partly a matter of choice.*

9. *I will always be able to learn something new.*

If you are ready to put the aging process ''on hold,'' move on to Chapter Two.

CHAPTER 2

The Elimination of Chronic Fatigue Helps Maintain Youth

Chronic fatigue will make a person feel prematurely old faster than almost any other single factor. But the good news is that it can be virtually eliminated. This chapter discusses the causes of chronic fatigue and the mechanisms by which it can accelerate the aging process. Following that, dietary guidelines and lifestyle changes which can be used to completely eliminate chronic fatigue will be detailed.

NOTE: There is a disease process called, among other things, the Epstein-Barr syndrome, which produces symptoms of chronic fatigue. It will be discussed later in this chapter. The current discussion concerns the chronic fatigue that is produced by the *lifestyles* that some individuals adopt.

What are the signs of chronic fatigue?

It is easy to spot a person who is chronically fatigued. He might as well be carrying around a sign that says "I'm always tired." His shoulders droop, the curvature of his spine is exaggerated, his abdomen pushes forward, his eyelids make feeble attempts to stay open, his chin protrudes weakly forward, and when he walks he shuffles along with obvious effort. He frequently experiences eyestrain, colds, and headaches, and is often handicapped by fuzzy thinking at the very time when he needs to be an alert, incisive decision maker.

Do we just run out of physical energy because we are on the job eight to ten or more hours a day? Do we experience chronic fatigue because we use up all of our glucose—that basic energy molecule which we obtain from the food that we digest and from the glycogen that is stored in our bodies? Depletion of energy stores is a factor in the production and maintenance of chronic fatigue, but it is not the only one. In fact, it is a minor one, because glycogen depletion is a condition which can be easily overcome. Chronic fatigue is a much more complex process than simply one of depletion of our available energy stores.

Is chronic fatigue really all that important?

Sometimes I don't think we take chronic fatigue as seriously as we should. Often when someone is chronically fatigued, we tend to shrug it off as being caused by his habit of "overdoing it." If he isn't the type to "overdo it," we chalk it up to laziness. Yet this complaint is one of the most common ones physicians hear from their patients.

Physicians are beginning to pay more attention when a patient says, "Doc, I'm always tired," because chronic fatigue significantly affects the lifestyles of individuals. The degree of impairment produced by chronic fatigue can be comparable to that of some serious, chronic diseases.

What causes chronic fatigue?

Several factors combine to bring on the syndrome of chronic fatigue:

The transmission of impulses by nerve cells requires energy. Repetitive transmission of these impulses, together with a less-than-optimal oxygen supply and a dwindling reserve of glucose will result in fatigue of the nerve cells.

Continuous muscle contraction, whether caused by physical activity or by tenseness, requires energy and will cause muscle fatigue.

Even a minimal reduction in the oxygen supply to the cells of the body will enhance the condition of perpetual tiredness.

Loading the body with chemicals—alcohol or other drugs—which the body was not designed to handle brings on chronic fatigue.

Glycogen depletion from the cells of the body, together with widely fluctuating blood levels of glucose, will promote a continual state of malaise and a feeling of "letdown" long before the day is over.

Let us begin our analysis of chronic fatigue by examining each of the above factors which cause it. Then we will consider the mechanisms whereby chronic fatigue could accelerate the aging process; describe an experiment which, if followed for the prescribed time, will give you striking, firsthand evidence of the way dietary habits can either promote chronic fatigue or help to eliminate it; and, finally, we will turn to specific dietary guidelines which can be used to *eliminate* chronic fatigue.

What are the factors that cause chronic fatigue?

Factor one: Fatigue of the nervous system. There are billions of individual nerve cells inside the brain and inside the large nerves of the body. If you could look inside the brain, you would see all those cells connecting the different parts of the brain to each other. Similarly, if you could look inside a large nerve in the arm, or in the leg, or in some other part of the body, you would find that it, too, is composed of many, many individual nerve cells. If the individual nerve cells do not function properly, there can be no "thinking," and there can be no signals sent to the muscles or other organs of the body to assist them in performing the functions which they were designed to perform.

During the process of thinking, impulses travel across many different nerves in the brain. If this is done repetitively for a sufficient period of time, those nerve cells will become fatigued. Trying to concentrate on one problem while simultaneously thinking about a thousand other things will hasten that fatigue.

If a nerve cell conducts an excessive number of impulses and/or becomes more metabolically active than usual, it might run out of energy. A nerve cell's function will be compromised if it is conducting the normal number of impulses, but is in short supply of either oxygen or glucose. These are probably the most common causes of nerve cell fatigue.

One study gives evidence that anxiety and depression may be linked to chronic fatigue (Kroenke, et al, *Journal of the American Medical Association,* 1988). Approximately one of four (24 percent) of the 1,159 adults surveyed identified fatigue as a major problem. Kroenke and his colleagues studied 102 subjects who had had chronic fatigue for at least 30 days and who had no other apparent illness. According to the psychological tests which the scientists administered, 82 of the subjects (80 percent) suffered from anxiety, depression, or both. By way of comparison, in a group of subjects who had suffered no chronic fatigue, only 12 percent showed abnormal levels of anxiety or depression.

While a study of this type doesn't *prove* a cause-and-effect relationship between anxiety or depression and chronic fatigue, it certainly indicates that such a relationship might exist, especially when it is possible to offer a reasonable physiological explanation for the mechanisms responsible. A chronic fear of things to come and a chronic present-moment despondency would make the most mentally strong person falter.

If the nerve cells in the brain become fatigued, an individual's thinking might become erratic, he might become drowsy, or he might just feel "numb" and unable to concentrate. If the nerve cells which supply the muscles become fatigued, this might cause trembling of the hands and jerky, shaky movements.

Some people seem to have the capacity to do mental "work" for prolonged periods of time without becoming tired. They are invariably at the forefront of their fields. Are they able to do more mental work because they know some secret, or because they have some unusual physical and mental abilities that other individuals don't have? No, that's highly unlikely. Why then is it possible for them to remain alert and mentally energetic long after the nervous system of an "ordinary person" becomes numb? Since the most probable cause of nerve cell fatigue is a reduction in the *optimal* oxygen and fuel supply to the nerve cells, the people with the capacity to do prolonged mental work have learned to prevent this reduction. We will see how anyone can learn to do this. If impulse conduction and increased metabolic activity cause nerve cells to use energy faster than that energy can be supplied, the cells will tire. Nerve cells obtain energy from glucose. If a relatively constant blood level of glucose can be maintained along with a constant supply of oxygen so that the glucose can be utilized, then there will be a ready supply of energy. The proper dietary plan can produce this outcome.

Nerve cells must have oxygen to survive and function. If nerve cells are deprived of oxygen for just *a few minutes*, they will die. If there is a slight reduction in the amount of oxygen supplied to nerve cells, their function will be compromised. Because the nerve cells are so sensitive to oxygen, and because they have such a critical need for it, the cardiovascular system is designed to allow a preferential blood flow to the nerve cells, even if blood flow to some other areas of the body must be curtailed. In the event of blood loss or other emergency, the cardiovascular system will make every effort to ensure that the brain gets an adequate supply of oxygen, even if other organs are deprived.

Factor two: Fatigue of the muscular system. The contraction of a muscle usually (but not always) results in the movement of the structure to which the muscle is attached. If the biceps, the muscle on the front of the arm, contracts, it will move the forearm because it is attached to the forearm. Because the biceps is capable of contracting, you are able to touch your chin with your hand. Movements of this nature require energy.

Energy is required for all muscular contractions. If you take a few hundred steps, enough to cover the distance of one mile, approximately 100 calories of energy will be required. Movement of the hands, arms, and legs requires energy; the contraction of the heart muscle to propel blood to the body requires energy; and the contraction of the muscles in the intestinal wall to aid the process of digestion requires energy.

Muscles use energy even if they don't produce movement when they contract. If you push on a wall, your muscles will require energy. The wall won't move, but your muscles will use energy when you push on it.

Muscular contraction causing the muscles to shorten and produce movement is known as *isotonic contraction*. Muscular contraction that does not result in a shortening of the muscles and does not produce movement is known as *isometric contraction*. Both types of contraction require energy, and both are used in normal daily activities. Isotonic contraction is necessary for actions such as walking, and isometric contraction for functions such as standing or sitting erect. Muscle tenseness, which is usually an unnecessary isometric muscular contraction, requires energy.

Daily fatigue can be prevented if the body has an adequate supply of glycogen. One might draw the conclusion that since muscle contraction (whether for purposes of movement, sitting erect, or from tenseness) requires energy, the muscles eventually use up all of their glycogen and chronic fatigue results. That is partially correct. Prolonged muscular contraction will eventually use up all of the stored glycogen, but that is not the likely cause of the chronic day-in-and-day-out fatigue that many of us experience. Normally the body is quite capable of storing almost any amount of glycogen that might be required for prolonged activity, certainly more than enough to keep an individual energized through an ordinary workday.

An example of the extent to which the body can store energy is the Ironman Triathlon held in Hawaii. The participants swim 2.4 miles in the ocean, climb out of the water and race 112 miles on a bicycle, then run a 26.2-mile marathon. Both men and women participate in this event. Some athletes have completed all three events in less than 10 hours.

Imagine an equivalent event in your life. Think of a friend or relative who lives approximately 100 miles from you. Visualize yourself getting on a bicycle and riding to see your friend. When you get there, you get off your bike and swim across a lake that is about two miles wide. (You know how long it takes you to *walk* two miles, but think about swimming that distance.) When you reach the other side of the lake, you see some runners getting ready to run a 26.2 mile marathon. You put on your running shoes and run the marathon with them. Incredible? Yes, it's incredible, but now you are beginning to get an appreciation of the capacity of the human body to store energy. If the human body can store enough glycogen to get individuals through a feat such as the Ironman Triathlon, it can certainly store enough so that glycogen depletion is not a significant factor in the production of chronic fatigue. Appropriate diet and aerobic activity can enable your body to store enough energy to keep you active and alert through a long day.

Factor three: Reduction of oxygen supply to the cells. The heart pumps blood to all parts of the body. The blood carries vitamins, minerals, and nutrients to the various tissues of the body. The blood also carries an element which is vital to our very existence: oxygen. More specifically, red blood cells carry oxygen to the tissues. When our oxygen supply is reduced, we function poorly, and without oxygen we cannot survive.

For optimum delivery of oxygen to the tissues, several conditions must be met: the blood must be able to flow easily to the tissues; the blood must contain a sufficient number of red blood cells; the red blood cells must contain a sufficient number of hemoglobin molecules; there must be an adequate amount of oxygen in the air which is inhaled; the inhaled oxygen must be able to pass from the lungs into the red blood cells; and, once inside the red blood cells, the oxygen must be able to bind to the hemoglobin molecules. If one or more of these conditions is not met, the flow of oxygen to the tissues may not be adequate for sufficient energy production. Reduced energy production will enhance the condition of chronic fatigue. Several of these conditions can change on a day-to-day basis.

If we are healthy and have an adequate intake of iron, we probably have a sufficient number of red blood cells and enough hemoglobin to transport the oxygen. The amount of oxygen in the air that we breathe may vary from day to day, depending on the conditions of crowding and ventilation in our work and play areas. The ability of oxygen to pass from the lungs into the blood probably doesn't change from day to day. It occurs easily unless there is chronic lung disease present. (A person who has chronic lung disease may help the process of oxygen transfer to the blood through breathing exercises and a program of physical activity.) Since the above conditions remain reasonably constant from day to day, that leaves two critical conditions which *can* change on a day-to-day basis (but which can be controlled). They are: (1) the ability of blood to flow to the tissues of the body, and (2) the ability of oxygen to bind to the hemoglobin molecules inside the red blood cells.

Factor four: The ablility of blood to flow to the tissues of the body. Here's how these changes occur: Blood consists of a watery substance (plasma) in which blood cells, nutrients, and other materials are suspended. If the blood is thin (has a low viscosity) and the blood cells are spaced apart, the blood will flow easily through the small blood vessels (capillaries) to the tissues of the body. Conversely, if the blood is thick (has a high viscosity) and the blood cells are clumped together, it will not flow as easily through the capillaries. If a person eats a meal which contains a lot of fat, the fat will be quickly absorbed into the blood. The fat which is eaten is not actually broken down in the digestive system, but is emulsified into small droplets. These droplets are absorbed and dumped directly into the bloodstream. When that happens, the change in the blood is so striking it can be seen with the naked eye. If a test tube full of blood is centrifuged, the blood cells go to the bottom of the tube, and the fluid part, or plasma, remains on top. Plasma which does not contain fat is clear, like water. Plasma which contains fat is cloudy and may be almost opaque because of the emulsified fat.

The fat in the blood makes the blood thicker and tends to make the red blood cells clump together. Both of these effects impede the oxygen delivery to the tissues of the body. The thicker blood flows more slowly through the blood vessels. Also, red blood cells are supposed to go through the capillaries in single file so that they can quickly and efficiently deliver oxygen to the tissues (and pick up carbon dioxide to be carried back to the lungs to be exhaled). Red blood cells that are clumped together obviously can't go through the capillaries single file. This causes a reduction in the amount of oxygen delivered to the tissues. Therefore the individual who eats a fatty meal in the middle of the day is going to compromise the delivery of oxygen to his tissues for the remainder of the day.

If the blood remains thin and the red blood cells don't clump together because of the presence of fat in the blood, the delivery of oxygen to the tissues will be efficient—that is, if the oxygen can freely bind to the hemoglobin. Very small quantities of carbon monoxide can inhibit that binding.

Factor five: The ability of oxygen to bind to the hemoglobin molecule. Carbon monoxide is present in smoke and may be present in polluted air. Carbon monoxide binds to the hemoglobin molecule at the same point on the molecule as does oxygen. What makes the situation dangerous is that carbon monoxide binds with more than 200 times the tenacity of oxygen. A small carbon monoxide pressure in the lungs—200 times less than that of oxygen—will cause half of the hemoglobin in the blood to become bound with carbon monoxide instead of with oxygen. The hemoglobin so bound will be unable to transport oxygen. If you work in an area that is polluted with smoke or other substances which contain carbon monoxide, the ability of oxygen to combine with the hemoglobin in your blood might well be compromised.

It is evident that a reduction in the oxygen supply to the cells of your body can help bring on chronic fatigue and that high blood-fat levels and exposure to carbon monoxide can reduce the delivery of oxygen to the tissues of your body.

Factor six: Adding chemicals to the body which it is not designed to use. The human body operates most efficiently on nutritious food and drink. Any chemical or compound which doesn't fall into that category is a substance that the body was not designed to use. The body can get rid of foreign substances (and detoxify certain poisonous agents), but that doesn't mean that the body was designed to *use* those substances. Humans consume an amazing quantity of pills, potions, supplements, and megavitamins, as well as over-the-counter drugs for headaches, weight control, colds, allergies, and other aches and pains. The body must detoxify, excrete, and/or inactivate all of these substances. Three of the most common chemicals which humans add to their bodies on a chronic basis are nicotine, alcohol, and tranquilizers.

Alcohol can contribute to chronic fatigue because it must be metabolized by the body and because, when it enters the bloodstream, it goes to the brain cells, where it acts as a sedative. Alcohol reacts at the same molecular sites on the nerve cells as do Valium and other sedatives *(FASEB Newsletter*, Vol. 20, No. 9, September, 1987).

Most alcoholic beverages contain some impurities—chemicals such as indols and skatols. These add to the early morning "mind fog." Also, alcohol causes the body to lose fluid by inhibiting one of the hormones (antidiuretic hormone) of the body. The sedative effect, the impurities in the alcohol, and the fluid loss, all contribute to the "hangover" or dull feeling that occurs following alcohol consumption.

Tranquilizers are a bit different. They can be both psychologically addicting because of the pleasure the drugs provide, and physically addicting because the brain eventually accepts them as a part of the normal brain chemistry. An individual only becomes aware of this when he tries to stop taking the drug. When that happens, the brain sends out a message which gives the person an enormous craving for the drug. Many individuals find it difficult to quit taking a drug that has both sedative and pleasure-producing components.

Adding chemicals to the body which are not nutritious, and which the body is not designed to use, will enhance the condition of chronic fatigue.

Factor seven: Fluctuating blood-glucose levels. Since the body metabolizes glucose in order to obtain energy, it is extremely important that the blood glucose levels be maintained in a relatively constant supply. This makes it possible for the body to transfer energy (in the form of glucose) from one part of the body to another.

If the muscles become active and begin to use large quantities of glucose, the blood-glucose concentration will begin to fall. The fall in blood-glucose concentration will stimulate the liver to release large quantities of glucose into the blood. This is the manner in which glucose is shifted from the liver to the blood to the muscles. The glucose in the blood can act as a highly responsive medium for the exchange of glucose from one part of the body to another.

Perhaps a more important reason for maintaining blood glucose at a constant level is that the rate of glucose transport to the brain is dependent upon the blood-glucose concentration. When the blood-glucose concentration falls, the availability of glucose to the brain decreases.

Since the brain derives essentially all of its energy from the metabolism of glucose, if the blood-glucose level falls to very low values, the metabolism of the brain will be depressed. For that reason, it is desirable that the blood-glucose levels be maintained at values that are near normal, and that they not be allowed to fluctuate severely during the day.

If attention is not paid to the ingestion of the proper quantity *and quality* of carbohydrates, the following cycle could develop: a person might ingest carbohydrates which can be quickly absorbed (such as the sugars which are found in candies and other sweets). This will cause the blood-glucose level to rise from 90 milligrams percent to 140 milligrams percent or above. The rise in the blood level of glucose will stimulate the pancreas to secrete insulin. The increased amount of insulin in the blood will bring the blood glucose not only back to the original level of 90 milligrams percent, but to a level lower than 90 milligrams percent—perhaps to 70 to 80 milligrams percent. This results in a feeling of malaise, letdown, and hunger, prompting the person to ingest additional simple carbohydrates which can be quickly absorbed and which will again raise the blood glucose levels above 140 milligrams percent. The cycle repeats itself.

Chronic fatigue stresses the body, and it is this stress which accelerates the aging process. When the body is continually stressed, a predictable sequence of events occurs, beginning in the brain.

How exactly does stress accelerate the aging process?

Stress causes the brain to release a hormone with the cumbersome name of "corticotropin-releasing factor," or simply CRF. The CRF, through a series of steps, causes another hormone, cortisol, to be released into the bloodstream. The cortisol causes the breakdown of complex, stored sugars, and the breakdown of tissue proteins. It also causes a decrease in the number of certain types of white blood cells. These changes make it more difficult for the body to fight diseases, allergies, and infections.

If stress continues for prolonged periods, cortisol will continue to be released into the bloodstream. The adrenal glands—glands which sit on top of the kidneys and produce the cortisol—will become enlarged. Other key organs, such as the thymus gland, the lymph nodes, and the spleen, will atrophy. When they shrink, the function of the immune system is impaired.

Does impairment of the immune system speed the aging process?

Yes. Scientists who study the aging process believe that a healthy immune system is essential. The immune system manufactures antibodies to protect us against foreign invaders, but as it loses its viability, it will gradually turn on the cells of the body. (This process is enhanced when the cells of the body change, and chronic fatigue speeds that process.) As the immune system attacks more and more cells of the body, the aging process becomes more and more evident.

So, now that you know that eliminating chronic fatigue will reduce chronic stress and thereby help prevent premature aging, you may be saying to yourself, "Good. You tell me to eliminate chronic fatigue and slow down the aging process. That sounds fine, but *how* do I eliminate chronic fatigue? *Saying* that it should be done and *doing* it are two different things. I have a (business, profession, family, whatever) to run. If I don't drive myself to the point of collapse, it won't get done." It may be somewhat easier to talk about eliminating chronic fatigue than to do it. . . but not much. If you would like to eliminate chronic fatigue and do *more* for your (business, profession, family, whatever) than you have been able to do in the past, read on.

Your body is a finely tuned machine. The fuel it uses will influence its performance on both a short-term and a long-term basis. Stoking your engines with the wrong fuel increases your chances of having heart disease, obesity, diabetes, cancer, arthritis, and other degenerative diseases. It affects the delivery of oxygen to the tissues; it can hasten the fatigue of nerve, muscle, and other body cells; and it can promote chronic malaise and letdown. Perhaps an examination of the two lifestyles described below will give you incentive to seek out quality foods for your system. If you have heart and blood vessel disease, if you have arthritis or some other degenerative disease, or if you have some condition that could be made worse by temporarily altering the delivery of oxygen to your tissues, don't *purposely* try to get chronic fatigue (just to see what it feels like) by following the first lifestyle described below. On the other hand, you might find, to your surprise, that you have been living this particular fatigue-producing lifestyle even though you have some of the above conditions. (Also, if you have a lot of work to do, or if you need to be unusually alert, don't try the fatigue-producing lifestyle just to see what it feels like.)

How do you get chronic fatigue?

Becoming chronically fatigued can be a completely painless process. It is possible that you have been in that state for years and have come to think of it as normal. Perhaps it's been a long time since you have experienced the exhilarating feeling that comes with having an energized body. It could be that you have been living the fatigue-producing lifestyle described below. If you haven't, and you're curious about how it feels, here's how to develop chronic fatigue:

1. Have a few cocktails this evening before dinner. (If you don't drink alcoholic beverages, eat something—candy or similar food—that contains a lot of sugar before dinner.) For dinner, eat beef, lamb, pork or other foods which have a high fat content. Almost anything that is fried contains a lot of fat. Have a dessert that contains a lot of sugar.

2. When you get out of bed in the morning, don't do any type of aerobic exercise such as walking, jogging, or riding a bicycle. Don't engage in any type of aerobic activity during the day.

3. For breakfast, have ham, eggs, and buttered toast, or a breakfast with an equally high fat content (omelets, French toast, fried foods).

4. At 10 a.m. eat a candy bar or some other food which contains a lot of sugar.

5. For lunch, have a glass of wine and a piece of pizza (or a Reuben sandwich, or similar food with a high fat content.) If you are in a hurry to eat lunch, eat a hamburger which contains two meat patties, cheese and "the works." That will give you *29 grams of fat* for lunch (even if you leave off the French fries and the milk shake.)

6. At 3 p.m. (if you are still awake) eat another candy bar.

7. In the evening, have a few cocktails, a steak for dinner, and a high-calorie, high sugar-content dessert.

Repeat the above seven steps for several days.

Did you feel sluggish, or did you feel energized? Did you feel lethargic, or did you feel supercharged? Did you feel alert and on top of every situation, or did you feel fuzzy and unable to follow all of the trains of thought?

If the process of becoming chronically fatigued described above sounds like a pretty ordinary way of life, that isn't too surprising. That is the way millions of people treat their magnificent human machines every day. As incredible as it might seem, a huge segment of the U.S. population has been in a state of chronic fatigue for years and thinks that it is normal; they think that everyone feels that way. Many will remain chronically fatigued permanently.

How do you get rid of chronic fatigue?

Now that you know how to bring on chronic fatigue, are you ready to get rid of it for good? If the seven steps described above will bring on the condition, won't taking opposite actions probably eliminate it? As a matter of fact, yes.

Following the steps outlined below will eliminate the fatigue. It will charge you with energy. If you aren't already living this type of lifestyle and want to see what it feels like to follow the steps for a few days, do it during a period when you have plenty of things to do. Otherwise you might find yourself with such a supply of excess energy that you will start to "bug" those around you.

During the time that you follow the steps, you won't be dumping a load of fat into your bloodstream. Blood will be flowing more freely to the tissues of your body. Your blood glucose will remain more constant (allowing your body to shift glucose to any cell in your body which has an immediate need for it). You will be more alert. You will have sufficient energy to carry you through to the end of a very long day.

Here's how to get rid of chronic fatigue:

1. Before dinner, instead of having an alcoholic beverage or snacks that contain sugar, have a "cocktail" of mineral water and fruit juice. The drink can be made in various ways. It can be made by combining chilled mineral water with orange juice or with lemon juice (but be creative with your own combinations). For dinner have two or three ounces of broiled fish or chicken (skinless), two green vegetables, and a complex carbohydrate such as a baked potato, brown rice, or pasta. For dessert, have some "ice cream." Make the ice cream by placing two frozen fruits (bananas and pineapple or other combinations) in a blender and blending until smooth. You will be alert during the remainder of the evening, and you will sleep well.

2. When you get out of bed in the morning, engage in 20 minutes of aerobic exercise such as walking, jogging, or bike riding. (If it is not possible for you to do this in the early morning, make it a point to get in at least 20 minutes of aerobic exercise sometime during the day.)

3. For breakfast, eat some fruit (grapefruit, orange slices, etc.) and high-fiber cereal with skimmed milk.

4. At 10 a.m. if you have a desire to eat something, eat a small apple, a peach, or 1/4 cup of raisins.

5. For lunch, have a complex carbohydrate (baked potato, small helping of rice, or pasta), and a green vegetable. Have a midday "cocktail" of mineral water and fruit juice.

6. At 3 p.m. if you can slow down long enough and if you want to eat, have something that contains a complex carbohydrate (apple, peach, banana, or raisins.)

7. In the evening before dinner, have a nonalcoholic hot apple toddy made with unsweetened apple juice.

Can chronic fatigue be permanently eliminated?

In order to shed the yoke of chronic fatigue permanently, repeat the above seven steps daily. Eat a variety of foods but make sure they are low in fat. For example, for breakfast a good choice would be whole wheat toast (with low-fat butter or butter substitute). For lunch, instead of the foods mentioned above, you could have a bowl of vegetable soup, a whole wheat roll, and a fruit cup for dessert. Use your imagination. There are many delicious foods which are nutritious and low in fat.

If you are chronically fatigued, switching to the lifestyle described above will make a *dramatic* difference in the way you feel. Your body will respond to what you feed it.

How specifically do the two lifestyles compare?

Specifically, one produces chronic fatigue, the other, boundless energy. If you were living the fatigue-producing lifestyle, the cocktails before dinner forced your body to contend with the sedative effect, the impurities, and the dehydrating effect of the alcohol. That's not all that your body had to contend with that evening.

The main course of your dinner was high in fat, and the dessert contained a lot of sugar. The fat in your blood caused your circulation to be sluggish and the red blood cells to clump together and hindered the supply of oxygen to your tissues as you slept. The sugar in the dessert, together with the alcohol, forced your body to contend with a high blood-sugar level (and the elevated blood insulin level that the high blood-sugar causes.) It's little wonder you weren't exactly ready to "take on the world" the next morning.

When you got out of bed the next morning, you not only didn't give your sluggish circulation a boost with some physical exercise, you gave it an additional challenge. The breakfast of ham, eggs, or other high-fat foods sent the blood-fat levels soaring again. Because of the seepage of fat from your intestine into your blood following breakfast, your blood again became thicker, the red cells again had an increased tendency to clump together, and the delivery of oxygen to the tissues of your body was inhibited.

Your body was unable to use the fat from the breakfast food for energy right away. Fat must first be broken down to fatty acids and glycerol. Then the fatty acids and glycerol must undergo additional chemical transformations in order for the body to obtain energy from them. Your body first used the alcohol and sugar which was consumed the previous night for energy. Any calories which were consumed but not used for energy were converted to fat and stored.

Immediately after breakfast, your body began clearing your blood of the fat which had seeped into it. Just as it was getting that process underway, your body had to contend with another challenge: your blood glucose level jumped to more than 140 milligrams percent because of your 10 a.m. candy bar.

The hyperglycemia that your candy bar produced brought forth a surge of insulin from your pancreas. The insulin began lowering your blood glucose by causing the glucose to enter the cells of your body. It brought the blood glucose first down to normal levels, and then to levels which were below normal. As a matter of fact, you were just beginning to feel a hypoglycemic (low blood sugar) letdown when it was time for lunch.

The wine at lunch enhanced the tranquilizing effect, and all of the other effects, of the previous night's alcohol. The fat which was ingested at lunch caused, by the mechanisms described above, a continued inhibition of the delivery of oxygen to the tissues of your body. The combination of the wine, the food, and the sugar caused the blood-glucose level to soar once again, and brought on yet another outpouring of insulin. You were well on the way to being partially sedated before lunch was over.

By the time you had your 3 p.m. candy bar, your body had not even begun to recover from the alcohol, the fat, or the elevated blood glucose. The 3 p.m. candy bar raised the blood-glucose level once more. During the next few hours, your blood-glucose level rose, came back to normal, and was entering the hypoglycemic letdown level at about the time you were ready to have your before-dinner drinks.

The entire cycle repeated itself the next day. The repeating cycles placed stress on your body. Your body was never able to fully regain its equilibrium from the nutritional roller-coaster ride of the previous day.

(Remember, while all of these physiological and metabolic swings were taking place in your body, YOU were supposed to charge through an activity-filled day without developing chronic fatigue!)

What if we choose the "boundless energy" lifestyle?

If, however, you have chosen to follow the second lifestyle that was described, your body will be having quite a different experience. When you have a before-dinner cocktail of mineral water and fruit juice, your body will be partially compensated for the dehydration which normally occurs during daily activities. Your blood volume expands, and the flow of blood to the cells of your body becomes more efficient.

When your dinner—even the broiled meat—is low in fat, that helps the situation. The green vegetables provide vitamins and fiber. The complex carbohydrates (potato, rice, or pasta) provide your body with a steady supply of carbohydrate for energy, as does the "ice cream" made from frozen fruit. Your blood, which is not thickened by fat, can flow freely to the cells of your body, carrying with it an ample supply of oxygen and energy. You sleep well.

In the morning (or later in the day) the aerobic exercise gives your heart, blood vessels, and muscles a boost. The exercise increases your body's ability to store glycogen.

Your breakfast starts you on the way to having an adequate intake of fiber. It doesn't load your blood with fat and interfere with the flow of oxygen to the tissues of your body or produce a drastic swing in your blood-glucose level.

The fruit that you have at 10 a.m. helps to maintain a steady supply of glucose for the cells of your body, while at the same time preventing drastic up-and-down changes in your blood-glucose level. Because the carbohydrate comes from fruit and not a candy bar, there is a more gradual passage of glucose from your digestive tract into your bloodstream. This makes it possible for your blood to quickly transport glucose to any cell of your body, including your brain cells, where it may be needed.

When it is time for lunch, you are still alert and energetic, and the type of food that you have then helps to ensure that you will continue to feel that way for the remainder of the day. The mineral water and fruit juice helps offset the dehydration which normally occurs, the vegetables provide fiber plus a rich supply of vitamins, and the complex carbohydrate assures a steady source of energy. Since your lunch is low in fat, the flow of oxygen to the tissues of your body is not compromised.

You are nowhere near a hypoglycemic letdown when you have your 3 p.m. complex carbohydrate, nor are you anywhere near one at the end of the day. At the end of the day your blood is still "thin" because of the absence of fat. It is still flowing freely to the tissues of your body and carrying a good supply of oxygen and nutrition; consequently, your body stores of glycogen have not been depleted, and your blood-glucose levels have not bounced up and down all day long. Each day that you live this way you will continue the process of revitalizing the cells of your body.

Have you ever wondered how someone like Artur Rubinstein could, at the age of 89, give one of his greatest performances ever at New York's Carnegie Hall? Have you ever wondered where individuals like Lee Iacocca of Chrysler or T. Boone Pickens of Mesa Petroleum get their drive and stamina? Do they know some "secret" that the rest of us don't know? Were they just born that way? Not likely. The dazzling achievements that they have enjoyed probably would not have been possible had they spent their days dragging around in a state of chronic fatigue.

NOTE: The chronic fatigue being considered in this chapter is the type that we bring on ourselves because of a partcular lifestyle, *not* the illness variously known as Epstein-Barr virus, "yuppie flu," or—the more recent label—"Chronic Fatigue Syndrome." Chronic Fatigue Syndrome consists of an overwhelming tiredness, tender lymph glands, sore throat, muscle aches, concentration difficulties, a "hungover" feeling, and depression. The syndrome isn't very common; it may occur in people who are eating right and getting plenty of rest, and it mimics the flu. There is no simple cure for ''Chronic Fatigue Syndrome.'' It may be treated with vitamins, aspirin for pain, exercise, and sleep to alleviate the symptoms. This type of treatment might cause remission, but the symptoms may persist despite treatment. Maybe we can't easily rid ourselves of ''Chronic Fatigue Syndrome,'' but we can rid ourselves of the plain old everyday chronic fatigue that is brought on by lifestyle.

Can chronic fatigue be effectively dealth with?

Chronic fatigue has such a devastating effect on the aging process that anyone who suffers from it and who wishes to look or feel younger than his chronological age, maintain his energy, alertness, vital thought processes, and creative capacities *must* deal with the syndrome. It should be exciting to learn that you *can* deal with it.

Aging occurs primarily because there is a reduction in the number of cells in the body and a reduction in the function of those cells which remain. Chronic fatigue contributes to both. The elimination of chronic fatigue slows both processes.

Nerve cells, for example, are lost each day. A reduction in the supply of oxygen and/or nutrients to nerve cells speeds their loss, thereby increasing the rate at which the nervous system ages. Long-term oxygen deprivation of any cells of the body will adversely affect the viability of those cells. Fluctuating blood-glucose levels may result in an irregular energy supply to the cells of the body, which will have a tendency to keep the metabolic machinery of the cells off balance.

As noted earlier in this chapter, the stress of chronic fatigue triggers the release of corticotropin-releasing factor (CRF) from the brain. CRF gears the body up to chronically repel the effects of stress. All of the systems of the body are affected, and all will age at a faster rate.

We will take a closer look at aerobics and nutrition later in this book. But for now, know that you *can* do something about eliminating chronic fatigue.

Summary

Begin now to inhibit the aging process by getting sound sleep at night. The nervous system recuperates and recharges its metabolic machinery during sleep. During sleep, provide your nervous system with a good flow of fat-free, well-oxygenated blood that contains a good supply of nutrients. When you awaken, your brain will be ready for some mental exercise. You will be alert, your thinking will be incisive, and you will be mentally energetic throughout a long day.

Begin now to inhibit the aging process by eliminating carbon monoxide from the air that you breathe. That will enhance the delivery of oxygen to the tissues of your body, and will enhance the viability of the cells of your body.

Begin now to inhibit the aging process by becoming more physically active. Physical activity, specifically aerobic activity, will increase the capacity of your body to store glycogen—that golden energy molecule. Remember, if individuals can store enough glycogen to complete the Ironman Triathlon, *you* can store enough glycogen to do almost *anything* that you want to do.

Begin now to inhibit the aging process by providing your body with steady intakes—small quantities, several times a day—of complex carbohydrates in order to give it a constant source of quality energy. Reduce your intake of fat so that fat contributes only 15 to 20 percent of your total calories. Increase your intake of fruits, green vegetables, and fiber-containing foods.

These few simple steps will provide the groundwork for your mental and physical metamorphoses into a new state of being. You will begin to shed your old skin. Your body will begin to heal from the bruises of past neglect. You will become alive with energy. You will say good-bye to chronic fatigue.

CHAPTER 3

Activating Your Brain Puts the Aging Process on Hold

Following a lecture that I gave on the effect of weight control and aerobic exercise on longevity, an individual brought up Sir Winston Churchill as an example of one whose lifestyle contradicted the concept that weight control and exercise are beneficial. Sir Winston, he said, was overweight, didn't exercise very much, was not averse to having a drink of Scotch, and chewed on cigars. Those statements are true, but Sir Winston had a phenomenally active mind. He kept his brain continually activated, and that, I am certain, was one of the things that put his aging process on hold. Before we go into a discussion of how to duplicate this feat, I would like to emphasize the value of protecting your brain from harmful substances such as carbon monoxide.

In Chapter Two you learned how to take better care of your brain. You learned that you could give it a steady supply of glucose by periodically eating foods which contain complex carbohydrates. You learned that you could enhance the flow of blood to your brain and to all of the other parts of your body, by eating less fat and keeping your blood "thin." You learned that you could increase the delivery of oxygen to your brain and to the other body tissues by not inhaling carbon monoxide, which ties up the oxygen-carrying molecules in your red blood cells. One of the prime sources of carbon monoxide is cigarette smoke.

What harm does cigarette smoking do?

Cigarette smoking increases the rate of hardening of the arteries (probably because the carbon monoxide in the smoke injures the cells which line the inside of the blood vessels).

Cigarette smoking also causes the small air sacs in the lungs (alveoli) to burst, producing the condition known as emphysema. The carbon monoxide in cigarette smoke significantly inhibits the delivery of oxygen to *all* of the tissues of the body. Therefore, if you want to eliminate these effects, *stop smoking*.

Easier said than done? Yes, but there is plenty of help available. If you fell out of a boat and couldn't swim, you wouldn't just give up—you would scream for help and you wouldn't be a bit embarrassed about it. If you smoke, you are also in a life-threatening situation, and if you can't make the necessary changes on your own, look for assistance. Many groups and organizations have programs that can help you stop smoking. Among them are Veterans Administration Hospitals, state health departments, and larger hospitals and medical centers. Contact one of them, or ask your physician to recommend a reputable program to you. Millions of people have stopped smoking and you can, too.

Now that you know how to provide your brain with the optimum supply of nutrition and oxygen, let us consider some of the methods of activating the brain and the benefits that result.

What makes some older people seem young?

Think of all of the people you know who act and look "young" even after they are well along in years. Don't they all have one thing in common? Aren't they all mentally active? Aren't they curious about the things around them? Aren't they alert, inquisitive, and involved with their occupations, hobbies, or other interests? Don't they pay attention to matters outside themselves? This mental activity seems to slow down the rate at which they age. It seems to pour a "life hormone," if you will, into their systems.

Allowing your brain the opportunity to be unusually active can produce that same "life hormone" for you. (You already know how to prevent chronic fatigue of your nervous system, now all you have to do is make it more active).

People who remain "young" even though their chronological age is advancing have learned to use their mental capacities efficiently. They don't unduly burden their brains with thoughts that have no relevance to the situation at hand. They generally don't worry about the things that they cannot change. More efficient use of the brain means that it can be used for longer periods of time and used more vigorously during those times.

How can I send the "stay young" message to my body?

Nerves regulate body function by innervating (attaching to) virtually every part of the body. They influence the function of every part of the body by causing the release of hormones which affect the body. If the brain and nerves are in a highly activated state, the message to the other systems of the body—to every single cell—is clear. That message is: "The body is in a state of high activity; and needs to remain alert, youthful, and energetic; there's no time to think about aging yet; it's all systems go." The brain, through the influence it exerts on the cells of the body and its hormonal systems, is a powerful controller of the body. The body responds to what the brain tells it.

How important is an active brain to remaining "young"?

Intense mental activity, an innate curiosity, and the feeling of having "one more thing to do" are the common features of prolonged youth that transcend race, sex, religion, culture, geographical areas and other individual differences. The object of the intense mental activity is unimportant—it can take the form of obsessive thinking about an occupation, of devotion to a hobby, or any other concern.

Formal education is not a prerequisite for mental activity. Henry Ford had only a very few years of formal education, no money, and no friends in high places, yet his achievements were notable. He was obviously capable of intense mental activity. Thomas Edison had no formal education, but he dreamed of a lamp that could be operated by electricity. He was able to bring that dream, as well as the dream of a dictating machine and countless other dreams, to fruition because he was capable of intense mental activity. A formal education may be helpful in obtaining certain objectives, but it certainly is not required for the kind of mental activity we are discussing.

In order to slow down the aging process, intense mental activity is essential. And remember: the healthier your body is, the more likely your brain is to be capable of this highly desired mental activity.

What role do the neurons play?

A neuron consists of a nerve cell body and all of its processes. The neuron has a cell body proper which contains all of the necessary metabolic machinery. This metabolic machinery utilizes glucose and oxygen to produce energy to carry on the day-to-day activities of the neuron. Nerve impulses are brought to the nerve cell body over structures called dendrites and are carried from the nerve cell body to other structures—muscles, glands, or other nerves—over structures called axons. Each neuron, then, is composed of dendrites, a cell body, and an axon.

Some neurons (sensory neurons) carry information (sensations such as touch) *to* the brain; others (association or connecting neurons) carry information from place to place *within* the brain and spinal cord; still others (motor neurons) that carry information *from* the brain and spinal cord to muscles, glands, and other parts of the body. There are billions of neurons in the nervous system.

Visualize for a moment one single, young, healthy, functioning neuron. What can you do to keep it that way forever? In essence, you can feed it, protect it from injury, and exercise it. That will keep it healthy all the way to the very end of your life span (approximately 110 years).

How can we feed our neurons?

With regard to feeding the neurons, we have already seen that the nervous system derives virtually all of its energy from glucose metabolism. Insulin is not necessary for that metabolism. The rate of glucose transfer into the brain is dependent on the concentration of glucose in the blood. When the blood-glucose level drops, the rate of transfer of glucose into the brain decreases, and brain metabolism is curtailed.

Brain metabolism is so sensitive to blood-glucose levels that if the concentration of blood glucose drops just a few percentage points, brain metabolism will be significantly curtailed. If the blood-glucose concentration drops from a normal level of approximately 90 milligrams percent down to 20 to 50 milligrams percent, convulsions and then loss of consciousness are likely to occur. It is important to maintain the blood-glucose level in the normal range. It was emphasized in Chapter 2 that the periodic ingestion of complex carbohydrates will help assure that the blood-glucose level does remain in the normal range. That will help one to remain alert and, at the same time, avoid the ''hypoglycemic letdown'' doldrums. If some individuals are able to remain mentally alert for longer periods of time than others, it may be that those individuals just have a different way of ''feeding'' their neurons.

Can we protect our neurons?

Visualize again that single, healthy neuron. How can you protect it from injury? First and foremost, maintain a good circulation of blood to your nervous system. Keep your blood flowing freely, keep it well oxygenated, and keep it "thin" by keeping the fat levels down. Neurons are sensitive not only to oxygen deprivation but to drugs, chemicals, and other agents which might pass from the blood into the brain. There is a "blood-brain barrier" that prevents some substances from entering the brain, but many substances *can* pass from the blood into the brain.

Anesthesia for surgery is possible because anesthetic agents can pass from the blood into the brain and alter the function of the neurons, thereby inducing a state of unconsciousness. Nicotine, caffeine, and alcohol can affect a person's mood because these substances cross the blood-brain barrier. A host of agents—drugs, chemicals, contaminants, pollutants—can pass from the bloodstream into the brain. The more you limit the number of "foreign" agents which get into your system and cross that barrier, the healthier your neurons will be.

Can we actually exercise our neurons?

Okay, your neuron is well nourished, it has plenty of oxygen, and it is free of chemical contaminants. Now all it needs is some exercise. Unfortunately, we adults all too often equate exercise with effort. We tend to be turned off to exercise—whether it's mental or physical—because when we think of exercise, the thought that "exercise equals effort" frequently flashes through our mind. It need not be that way. Many enjoyable activities—putting a puzzle together, painting a picture, building model ships—stimulate neurons and are fun besides. Trying something absolutely new just for the fun of it is wonderful exercise for your brain. If you have never planted a tulip, built a dollhouse, played a tune on a guitar, or any other of a number of things, that's wonderful. You have some things left to do that you haven't done before. Give some of them a try. You'll love doing them. Your flabby neurons will appreciate the refreshing change.

Aristotle supposedly said that the formation of habits is the basis of moral excellence. Habits may be fine some of the time, but living too much of your life through habit will deprive some of your neurons—perhaps your most creative ones—of the opportunity for exercise. Try changing some of your habits just for the purpose of neural stimulation.

The next time you cook something, alter the recipe or invent a new one. Go home from work by a different route, eat lunch at a different time, have fish instead of turkey for Thanksgiving, read *National Geographic* tonight instead of watching television. Habit-changing will stimulate your neurons, your nerves and whole body will begin to come alive, and you will begin to take on a younger, more radiant look. You will feel like walking down the street and seeing some of the world rather than lying on the couch with your feet propped up.

Is it a proven fact that looking forward to doing new things prolongs youth?

Yes. Here are some excerpts from an article by Susan G. Christensen in the April 1, 1990, *Clarion-Ledger* (Jackson, Mississippi) newspaper:

> Charity Drummond demonstrates how to stand up to old age.
>
> She squares her thin shoulders, thrusts out her chest and impertinently tilts her chin.
>
> She may be 98, but she's not folding. ''You don't want to hump over and say I'm old,'' says the petite bundle of bravado. ''I'm going to be at least 125.''
>
> Friends of the feisty Jackson woman figure it's no idle boast. When Drummond decides to do something, you best get out of her way.
>
> Consider:
>
> Drummond got her driver's license at age 72 because she was tired of waiting on rides.
>
> Ten years later, she climbed into a cockpit in Houston, Texas, to satisfy a lifelong desire ''to fly with the ducks and the buzzards.''
>
> ''The first time I went up, he (the teacher) had me land and it was as smooth as it could be. Not a bounce or anything. I wasn't scared not one bit. The teacher said, 'You're the only one I ever took up who was not nervous.'''
>
> ''I must have been a pilot in my other life.''
>
> Indeed, Drummond is rarely out of her dancing shoes. When she is not waltzing solo across her efficiency apartment at Madonna Manor in Jackson, she's playing belle of the ballroom at local veterans' clubs.

"They all want to dance with me because I dance *with* them. I don't jump up and down."

"She probably goes out more at night than anyone I know," says Madonna Manor manager Juanita Weatherford. "She seems more energetic than anyone else."

"I have to have something to do all the time. I have kits to put together. I play cards. I'm going to have to start piecing quilts. I have to keep busy."

No doubt about it—Charity Drummond is a living lesson on keeping the mind young. She stays busy and is always looking forward to doing something new.

The farmer who wants to plant one more crop, the grandparent who wants to get to know that next grandchild, the sports fan who wants to see how his team does next season, the businessman who is going to continue to operate one more year, the tourist who wants to travel to one more place, and the person who wants to watch the outcome of events in this or that part of world, all have one thing in common: they have a *purpose* for continuing. They are looking forward to one more situation and they just *have* to see it through. Their nervous systems are alert and alive and so they feel and look younger than they would if life held no purpose for them.

I read recently of a married couple, both in their early 90s, whose hobby is growing flowering plants. They graft orchids that will not produce flowers for *five years*. That pretty well settles the fact that they have to stay around for at least another five years to see how the flowers are going to turn out.

Are purpose and mental activity essential?

Yes, they are. Purpose and intense mental activity, discussed in the section above, go hand in hand. Purpose is that drive which keeps one going, and intense mental activity is the process which keeps the individual's neurons "in shape." Almost everyone possessed of purpose engages his mental faculties, thereby not only achieving an end result but reaping other benefits along the way.

It is now well established that altering certain physiological processes can increase the life span. Although the mechanism is not yet fully understood, it is highly likely that the brain can be influenced by several different stimuli to readjust its "aging clock" thereby lengthening the life span. It has been documented that food restriction (reduced intake of nutritious food—not malnutrition) can increase the life span of the experimental animal. Intense mental activity, a purpose for living, dietary manipulation, and other processes may very likely, if properly applied, increase the life span of humans.

But is it worth the effort to merely prolong our existence?

Yes, I definitely believe it is worth the effort. These manipulations do not simply prolong our existence, they *delay aging.* They stretch out our middle years. Manipulating the diet of experimental animals—even if begun when they are adults—*can delay aging and increase the life span by 30 to 40 percent.* If manipulating the diet of humans (together with continued mental activity and a purpose for living) increased life span by a significant amount as many scientists believe it can, then the vastness of the changes we would have to consider would be formidable. Would you retire at age 65 if you knew that you were going to live to be 110? Would you buy life insurance at age 30? Would you have children while in your 20s? Would you have a second career? At what age would you get married? What about all of the other timetables of society? The scope of the changes in our timetables may seem threatening to some people. I believe that these changes are inevitable.

Consider a hypothetical situation for a moment. Suppose it became an accepted way of life for each individual to have two careers before he retired. A person would, for example, enter the field of marketing at the age of 25. While pursuing a successful career in that field, he would spend some time preparing for a second career. Then after 25 years in marketing, he would, at the age of 50, take a few years for additional, concentrated study in preparation for his second career. He would then, say, become a history professor. He would follow that career for 20 years, retire at the age of 75, then devote his remaining 30 or so years to his avocation.

At the present time it is not possible to offer incontrovertible proof that stimuli such as purpose, intense mental activity, physical activity, or manipulation of food intake will increase the human life span by a specific number of years, but there are indications, based on studies done with human population groups and experimental animals, that these stimuli will prolong life to some degree. The fact that proof that a specific number of years can't be added to the life span doesn't mean that we should wait around before beginning to apply the principles.

We can begin to apply certain principles now, while studies on the aging process are being done. In some cases we don't have to wait 100 years to see if a particular lifestyle change is going to prevent premature aging. We can use biological markers to make that determination.

Certain body functions change with age. Kidney function, maximum oxygen consumption, reflexes, and other parameters change as individuals get older. These are biological markers that can be measured and used to determine a person's functional age (a person with a chronological age of 50 might turn out to have a functional age of 40). Once the biological markers have determined the functional age, measurements can be made again some years later to indicate whether a particular regimen is preventing premature aging. Thus the effect of a particular food, drug, lifestyle change, or other parameter on the aging process can be studied over a short span of time—perhaps five years—rather than over a lifetime.

What is cogitation and how important is it?

Cogitation is the capacity to think or reflect. Since activating the brain puts the aging process on hold, it is worth noting that cogitation is a very effective activator of the neurons in the brain. Many people go through numerous daily activities without having to cogitate at all—without having to "figure out" anything. They drive to work, eat lunch, talk to co-workers, perhaps even do their work, watch a movie, listen to music, cook dinner, clean house, and undertake other activities without having to cogitate to any significant degree.

If the performance of a task requires that you think with intensity and objectivity, you are cogitating. That type of thinking is frequently avoided because it requires effort. This well-known phenomenon is illustrated by the old story of the man whose job it was to bag potatoes for shipping. As potatoes of all sizes came down the conveyor belt, he had to take them off and place them in bags. He placed the large potatoes in one bag, the medium-sized potatoes in another bag, and the small ones in a third bag. When someone asked if it was hard work, he said that the work was easy, but that making the decisions was exhausting.

So it is with cogitation. Even though cogitation can put the neurons through their paces and can be fun, it does require some effort.

The very fact that it does require effort is the reason that it is so effective in activating the brain. That cogitation activates the neurons in the brain has been demonstrated in humans by using a process known as positron emission tomography (PET). PET makes possible the imaging of metabolic functions in the body, of "visualizing" chemical reactions. The image is formed by a computerized synthesis of data transmitted by positron-emitting substances that have been incorporated into natural biochemicals and given to the patient. Computer analysis of the data shows up as different colors (or the absence of colors); the colors or their absence represent the rate of metabolism (energy usage) in specific tissues.

Active areas in the brain can be "visualized" by using PET. The use of PET to study human subjects has shown some fascinating results. When volunteers performed mental tasks, the neurons in the brain became more active, but the area of the brain involved depended on the type of mental task undertaken. The area that became activated when subjects performed mathematical exercises was different from the one activated when they painted pictures. Different tasks required different sets of neurons. The implication is that cogitation on a variety of subjects activates more total neurons.

If you write a poem, redecorate a room, plan an event, or paint a picture, if you learn to play a musical instrument, to tune up an automobile, to take pictures with a new camera, to sew, to sail, to work with stained glass, or any number of other activities that can be fun, you are stimulating a multitude of neurons in your brain by the process of cogitation. You are prolonging the youth of your nervous system.

How can the mind focus on the activities at hand?

Let me give you one man's solution. William Osler was born in Canada. He claimed that he was an ordinary individual, that his talents were mediocre—and claimed that his intimate friends knew that his talents were mediocre. Be that as it may, he was an advocate of working in "day-tight" compartments. He looked upon a day as a compartment of time which a person could use effectively by simply concentrating on doing what needed to be done during that day. He looked neither backward to things which might have been left undone nor forward to things which were yet to be done. Osler further subdivided each day into "hour-tight" compartments. He concentrated intently on the business at hand during that one-hour compartment of time, without looking backward to the hour that had just passed or forward to the hour that had not yet arrived. He didn't work in a hurry-up, hustle-bustle fashion. He calmly and methodically directed his thoughts and efforts to the task at hand.

Osler first studied the arts, and later developed an interest in medicine. After he received his medical degree, he became a professor of medicine and was one of the founders of the Association of American Physicians. He became the first professor of medicine at the Johns Hopkins Medical School. Having helped transform medical education by bringing the teaching of medicine into the hospital wards, he became a professor of medicine at Oxford University and, at the age of 62, received a baronetcy. His textbook of medicine became one of the leading texts of its day.

Osler was often asked about his successful life. In an address to the students at Yale, he revealed the "secret" of his success, duly noting that because of the simplicity of the message, some would turn away and not heed it. His "secret" was to live in day-tight compartments *with the mind concentrating intently on the business at hand.*

Can "tight-compartment" thinking really help concentration?

There is no question that you can achieve a more intense level of activation of the mind if past and future events are shut out during the period of concentration. After your neurons have been vigorously exercised in this fashion, you can allow them a time for recovery. By so doing, you will be applying one of the basic mechanisms for imparting strength to any part of your body, namely: Exercise + Recovery = Strength.

Enjoying your *leisure* time in day-tight compartments can also be helpful in that regard. When you play, if you shut out thoughts of yesterday's events as well as those pertaining to tomorrow, you will be allowing the neurons which you exercised while working an ample opportunity to recover and gain strength. It does take practice to learn to work and play in day-tight compartments. But then, what have you ever learned to do that is really worthwhile that didn't take practice?

Summary

This is your moment of decision. Promise yourself that before you read any further in this book, you will determine what there is in your life that you can get really excited about. What do you truly enjoy and prefer doing more than anything else in the world?

If you can't think of anything, then try making a list of the things that you would like to do and have never done, but which you think you *can* do or *can learn* to do. You don't have to be lord of the admiralty or prime minister to get excited and involved in something. Select something from that list and take some steps immediately—right now, today—to begin.

People have said to me, "Oh, I would like to do this or that, but it would take me five years to learn to do it. In five years I'll be 35 (or 45, or 65, or 75) years old." If a similar thought crosses your mind, remind yourself that in five years you are going to be that old anyway. You are going to be older a year from now whether or not you pursue your interest, so why not pursue it? You might find that instead of simply being talented at what you elect to try, you are gifted at it. You might discover an interest that will keep you happy and engaged from now on. It is *essential* that you keep your brain activated in order to put your aging process on hold. Do it!

CHAPTER 4

Nutrition and Your Aging Clock

Sometimes when we're trying to do something, we overlook the basics. A friend of mine discovered this one day soon after he had purchased a sailboat. He had spent an afternoon sailing, had come into port, taken his boat out of the water, and strapped it to the trailer, all in proper nautical fashion. Then he raised the trailer off the ball of the bumper hitch and watched trailer, boat, and contents slide down the steep ramp to the watery depths, out of sight forever. . . . almost.

Unfortunately, the mast just would not go under, thereby allowing him to feign ignorance as to the whereabouts of the vessel and to conduct salvage operations secretly in the dead of night. To make matters worse, his wife's loud guffaws alerted nearby sailors to his plight.

His sailor friends, having experienced similar disasters themselves, hooted with laughter. While helping him retrieve his boat and offering plenty of friendly "counsel." They told him that a wonderfully clever device—a block of wood—had been developed to keep boat trailers on the ramp. It functioned best, they said, when placed immediately behind the wheel of the trailer. He never again forgot that basic item.

When and how can I start being younger and healthier?

Let's not overlook something very basic when we consider preventing premature aging: *we can start being healthier and slowing down the aging process today simply by eating the right foods.* If we begin getting the correct balance of proteins, fats, carbohydrates, vitamins, and minerals, we will immediately notice a difference in the way we feel. Our thinking will become clearer and our eyes brighter, and we will have more energy. When the cells of our bodies begin drinking in the nutrients of which they have been so long deprived, we will begin to look, feel, and act younger. We will immediately begin to inhibit any premature aging which is taking place in our body.

So much has been written about what people should or shouldn't eat that at times we might be tempted to throw up our hands and say, "Forget it. No one seems to know what I should or shouldn't eat. Everyone seems to have a different opinion. I'll just eat what I please until they can agree."

That attitude is understandable in view of the large number of opinions on nutrition, many of which are scientifically unfounded, which exist today.

Yet, in almost no other area of our culture has there been such an enormous accumulation of *scientifically valid* data—data which is directly applicable to humans for promoting better health, decreasing the incidence of degenerative diseases, extending life expectancy, and now, perhaps for the first time, even for extending life span. Since there is a significant amount of "data" in print which isn't valid, you might wonder whether it is possible to sort through the morass of information and decide for yourself which is acceptable. Unfortunately, there is no foolproof method for doing that. However, the following suggestions might be helpful:

How can I be sure the nutrition book I am using is safe?

First, check the credentials of the author. Some authors are well-trained, legitimate scientists. Others aren't. If the author claims to have a "doctorate," and you don't recognize the name of the institution from which he received his doctorate, closer scrutiny of his qualifications is appropriate.

The second thing that you can do if you are in doubt about some new data or some new information which an author is presenting is to discuss it with your physician. He might be the first to tell you that his education and training weren't perfect, but he *can* evaluate new data, and he *can* assess the validity of the source from which it came.

Third, beware of inflexible programs which demand that you eat certain foods at certain times of the day and finally, beware of programs which promote vitamins, pills, gimmicks, or name-brand foods and drinks. Let's examine some nutritional information about which a good deal is known.

Carbohydrates are the foods which are preferred by the cells of your body for the production of energy. If carbohydrates are not available, the cells will begin to use the glycogen which is stored in the body.

Glycogen is stored in the liver and to a lesser extent in the other body cells. As you use glycogen, your body loses water. The dehydration causes a temporary loss of body weight. As your body becomes depleted of glycogen, chronic fatigue may develop.

After all of the glycogen has been used, the cells of your body will begin to break down fat and protein for energy. By restricting your intake of carbohydrates, you force your body to break down the fat and protein. This is accomplished through a complex series of chemical reactions, known as gluconeogenesis, to supply the needed glucose to your cells for energy. Gluconeogenesis literally means the formation of "new" glucose, in that it is formed either from proteins or from the glycerol of fats. The process occurs in the liver.

Breaking down carbohydrates is a more efficient way of obtaining energy than breaking down fat and protein. But your body will get the glucose that it needs—if not from carbohydrates then from fat and protein.

How can my body convert fat and protein to glucose?

Your body can get glucose by converting stored fat to glycerol, which, in turn, can be converted to glucose. If the body must rely heavily on stored fat for energy, the fat may be incompletely broken down, causing the formation of substances in the blood called ketone bodies. As your body excretes the ketone bodies, additional water is lost, contributing to the dehydration which results from glycogen depletion. Carbohydrates are necessary both as an efficient energy source and for the fat-burning process. An adequate intake of carbohydrates prevents the adverse effects of improper fat metabolism.

If your body is not adequately supplied with carbohydrates, it can get glucose by converting protein to compounds called keto acids. The keto acids can then enter a chemical reaction cycle (the citric acid cycle) and produce energy. You need carbohydrates in order to maintain the tissue protein in your body. If your body must use protein for energy, it may obtain the protein from the liver, muscles, or other organs, including the heart.

If your body does use protein for energy, the first step in the breakdown of the protein is a process known as deamination. This is a reaction in which an amino acid is split to form a molecule of ammonia and a molecule of keto acid. The ammonia is converted to urea and is excreted in the urine. The keto acid enters the citric acid cycle to produce energy. This energy is transferred to the energy-bearing compound known as adenosine triphosphate, or simply ATP. The human body's ability to convert fat and protein to glucose is a mechanism that is built into the body to help ensure its survival. It isn't the most efficient way for the cells of the body to obtain glucose, but they can obtain it that way.

How can I build and maintain muscle?

If you could magnify one of your muscle cells 30,000 times (this is possible using an instrument called a transmission electron microscope), you would see a number of oval-shaped structures called mitochondria. All cells of the body contain mitochondria, and that is where energy that the cells use is produced. The more active cells of the body, such as muscle cells and liver cells, contain large numbers of mitochondria; less active cells contain fewer.

Carbohydrates are the "muscle-building" and muscle-maintaining foods and are the preferred energy source of the mitochondria. When day-to-day muscle activity increases, the number of mitochondria increases. It is said that "red meat builds muscle." I suspect this myth began simply because red meat is muscle, and it was easy to believe that ingested meat was converted to muscle inside the human body. Red meat contains protein and a lot of fat. The body can, through a series of complex chemical processes, break down and convert both protein and fat into molecules which can be be used for energy by the muscles. However, that is not the best way to build and maintain muscles. If your intake of protein is sufficient (two to three ounces a day) to provide for the growth and repair of tissue, you can build muscles more efficiently by having the optimum intake of quality carbohydrates.

What do quality carbohydrates do?

We have already seen that glucose is essential for the proper functioning of the central nervous system. A constant supply of glucose, which comes from complex carbohydrates, will help prevent the fatigue, dizziness, headache, and hunger which accompany low blood-glucose levels.

How do carbohydrates slow the aging process?

Just as carbohydrates are the best foods for building and maintaining muscle cells and are essential for the proper functioning of nerve cells, so are they the best foods for maintaining the viability of other body cells. This is very important in slowing the aging process. Here's why: aging occurs primarily because of a decrease in the number of cells in the body and because of a decrease in the function of those cells which remain. That makes it imperative that the mitochondria within the cells of the body get the food they prefer to use to produce energy.

Plants use energy from the sun to combine carbon dioxide and water to produce carbohydrates. This process is known as photosynthesis, during which oxygen is also produced. Starch, the most common plant carbohydrate, is a complex compound of simple sugars. It is found in seeds, grains, beans, peas, corn, potatoes, and roots of vegetables. When you get your complex carbohydrates from plants, you also get essential vitamins, a multitude of minerals, many of the amino acids, plus another beneficial substance—fiber. About 50 percent of the calories in the average American diet comes from carbohydrates. This is much too low; we should be getting at least 70 percent of our calories that way.

Which carbohydrates are right for you?

Even the figure 50 percent is misleading. Approximately one-fourth of those carbohydrate calories comes from ordinary sugar (sucrose), instead of from complex plant starches. Sucrose contains no vitamins, minerals, or other essential elements, other than calories. Sucrose, a disaccharide, is quickly broken down in the digestive tract into two simple sugars called monosaccharides. The two monosaccharides derived from sucrose are rapidly absorbed into the bloodstream, as are simple sugars from other sources. The simple sugars quickly flood the system, and just as quickly disappear. In the process they cause the blood-insulin levels to "bounce" up and down.

The large carbohydrate molecules, such as the plant starches, cannot be absorbed into the bloodstream without first having been broken down to simple sugars by the digestive process. The starches are acted upon by enzymes found in saliva, by an enzyme from the pancreas and finally by intestinal enzymes before they are converted to simple sugars. The energy that the body derives from complex carbohydrates digested in this way is provided in a time-release fashion. Consequently, there is a constant, steady source of energy for the body. Because there is a steady absorption of simple sugars, as opposed to a rapid absorption, the blood-insulin levels don't bounce up and down as the energy needs of the body are being met.

If we adjust our diets so that at least *70 percent* of our calories comes from carbohydrates instead of the current 50 percent, our bodies will have an even better supply of quality energy.

The starches are not the only source of glucose; they are just the best source. When common table sugar, sucrose, is converted from a complex sugar (disaccharide) to two simple sugars (monosaccharides), the simple sugars which are formed are fructose and glucose. Fructose, in addition to being one of the breakdown products of table sugar, is found in fruit and honey. It can be used for energy by the body. When lactose, a complex sugar which is in milk, is broken down to two simple sugars, the simple sugars which are formed are galactose and glucose. Thus, starches, sucrose, and lactose all produce glucose as one of their breakdown products. For that reason, glucose represents about 80 percent of the final products of carbohydrate digestion.

What is the purpose of glucose?

Once glucose enters the cells of the body, it has only one purpose: to be chemically broken down to provide energy for an important compound that is essential for every single body function. That energy-bearing compound is called adenosine triphosphate, or ATP. ATP is a carrier of energy. When a cell of the body needs energy for muscle contraction, conduction of nerve impulses, digestion, tissue repair, or for any other purpose, the ATP delivers that energy. Chemical processes within the cells of the body must produce the energy for the ATP to carry around. The chemical transformation of glucose inside the cell provides that energy.

This is how that transformation takes place: Initially glucose is changed, by a series of more than a half-dozen chemical reactions, into a compound called pyruvic acid. In the process of forming the pyruvic acid, enough energy is provided to form two ATP molecules. The pyruvic acid then goes through a chemical cycle (called the citric acid cycle) and an electron transport process to form 34 additional ATP molecules. This can be summarized as follows: one glucose molecule can be chemically transformed to produce enough energy to form 36 energy-bearing ATP molecules.

Is there an elixir of youth?

There is no magical formula, but a quality source of energy is required to keep the human body active and in good health to the end of the 110-year life span. A quality source of energy is also required to help the human body maintain a youthful appearance and inhibit the aging process.

From the cradle to the grave, the human body undergoes continual adaptation. A quality energy source allows this adaptation to operate at peak efficiency. Just a change from one age to another (from childhood to puberty to adolescence) constitutes a certain natural "stress" to which the body must adjust. Years ago, the energy required for the adaptation to these changes was appropriately termed *adaptation energy* (Selye, 1956). If you have an abundance of adaptation energy, you will be healthier, stronger, younger, more resistant to disease, more active, more "alive," and more likely to make an uneventful journey across the span of time which is your life span.

This adaptation energy, energy of life, or whatever you choose to call it, is the nearest thing we have to an "elixir of youth." Several things appear to influence its presence; among them are goal seeking, expectations, mental and physical activity, and an ideal state of energy balance.

You are a goal-seeking organism. All humans are. Humans function best when they are moving forward rather than stagnating. In that respect, they are much like a bicycle. As long as a bicycle is moving forward, it glides along smoothly, in a well-balanced position. But let it stop, and it falls. When humans are moving forward, they are gliding along in a smooth, well-balanced position.   They are generating adaptation energy—that energy of life. Let them stop or stagnate, though, and they too will fall—usually both mentally and physically. The adaptation energy ceases to be produced at the former level. Energy—quality energy—is required for enthusiastic goal seeking.

The 90-year-old couple we met earlier were grafting some flowers which wouldn't produce blooms for another five years. Naturally they *have* to stay around to see how the flowers turn out. By further activating their subconscious mechanism for goal seeking, they have stimulated their bodies to produce additional adaptation energy. Let's see what you could do with an experiment in which you suppress the level of adaptation energy.

It would be a cruel experiment, but if you could *convince* a 40-year-old that he should take it easy because he is old, that he might as well give up mental pursuits of any kind because he is old, that he looks old, that he is becoming feeble, that he is forgetful, and that he looks sickly, he would *become* old within a few years. (Notice I said that he would *become* old, not that he would *think* that he is old.) Why would he become old? Because of a precipitous decrease in the energy of adaptation, or energy of life.

Don't we usually get what we expect?

Absolutely. Did you know that following surgery, some patients heal faster than others? Part of that is due to the patient's age and state of health, but a large part of it is due to the fact that some patients *expect* to get well soon. Expectation changes the level of hormones and other chemicals in the body. Optimistic expectation, like excitement, raises the level of the beta endorphins (endogenous morphines), other endorphins, and other chemicals in the blood. Expectation also raises the level of the energy of adaptation in the body. Mental and physical activity have the same effect. Let's examine another phenomenon which expectation influences.

Placebos are "sugar pills," or inert substances that a patient believes to be a medicine. Placebos often have beneficial effects on the patients who take them. These effects have been measured and scientifically verified. The only explanation for the beneficial effect of placebos is that the patient *expects* the "medicine" to do him some good. The expectation, in turn, changes the level of endorphins and other hormones and chemicals in the blood. The expectation changes the level of adaptation energy in the body of the patient who takes the placebo.

Why am I making such a point of all of this? Because I want to emphasize the importance of energy in the life process—not just the everyday energy required for muscle contraction, digestion, respiration, and all of the other body functions—but the energy of adaptation, the energy of life.

I want to emphasize to you the importance of having a ready supply of that life energy, in addition to having a ready supply of the energy which is required for all of the day-to-day functions of your body.

The correct combination of foods provides the body with a quality energy source. All of the foods, vitamins, and minerals are important, and it is important to consume them in the proper quantities—more is not necessarily better. Since complex carbohydrates are of paramount importance, they have been discussed first. It is also important to include fat and protein in the diet, but diets which contain too much fat and protein perpetuate conditions such as hypoglycemia and chronic fatigue.

What types of foods provide quality energy?

Raw vegetables and fruits which contain complex carbohydrates are particularly important. They are more likely to contain all of the essential vitamins and minerals. Salads, raw vegetables, and fresh fruits are such excellent sources of complex carbohydrates, vitamins, and minerals that they are almost a one-stop shop for your nutritional needs. Begin eating more raw fruits and vegetables today. That should immediately begin to make you look and feel younger.

It is necessary to cook some foods which contain complex carbohydrates so that they will be more palatable. Another reason for cooking such foods is that we can eat more of them that way, and it is difficult to eat enough raw foods every day to get the required number of calories. Does that statement really mean that we could nibble away on raw fruits and vegetables throughout the day without being concerned about taking aboard too many calories? Yes, we very probably could.

Expectation helps provide the energy of life. The overall goal of this book is to help you turn your body into a lively, pulsating bundle of energy, thereby helping you to inhibit the aging process on the different systems of your body. In that regard, all of the food elements are important. Let's continue the discussion of the basics of metabolism by examining the role of dietary fat in maintaining the body in an optimum state of health.

What is the purpose of fats in the diet?

Your body can break down (catabolize) fats to be used as energy, or it can synthesize (anabolize) fats from fatty acids and glycerol. Your body cari also convert excess carbohydrate and/or protein to fat.

Containing approximately twice as much energy per gram as either protein or carbohydrate, fat provides the body with a large store of reserve energy. Fat is easily transported and easily stored, but it isn't necessary to consume fat in order to have it available for storage. Any type of excess food can be converted to fat and stored.

Fat anabolism includes the synthesis of some vital compounds that your body needs in order to function at peak efficiency. These compounds include phospholipid, an important component of cell membranes, and 7-dehydrocholesterol, which is necessary for vitamin D production. Your body can synthesize certain fatty acids—the saturated ones—but others, particularly the unsaturated fatty acids, *must be provided by the diet.* The ones so provided are known as *essential fatty acids,* and your body must have them. They produce such important compounds as the prostaglandins.

Prostaglandins are a group of biologically active lipids (fats). This exciting group of compounds was first discovered in the 1930s, but only in recent years has their critical importance to the body been fully recognized. The prostaglandins in your body serve a number of functions. They can be thought of as "tissue hormones." They are often produced within a particular tissue and travel only a short distance to act on the cells of that tissue. They have been identified in the reproductive organs, lungs, eyes, kidneys, brain, and in the organs of the immune system. They are among the most potent of all biological compounds.

If your body has the essential fatty acids that it needs to produce the prostaglandins, the function of many of your systems will be enhanced. The prostaglandins affect blood pressure and are important for certain gastrointestinal and metabolic functions, for intestinal motility, and for the regulation of acid production by the stomach. They also play an important role in the reproductive system.

The prostaglandins are found in almost every tissue of the body. A great deal of basic biologic information is yet to be gained by studying them. The potential therapeutic use of prostaglandins is enormous. Studies of these substances, which are capable of regulating hormone activity at the cellular level, constitute exciting new areas of medical research which will allow an understanding of many diverse disease processes and body functions.

In order for you to keep these ''tissue hormones'' active in virtually every part of your body, a supply of essential fatty acids is necessary. Your body can convert carbohydrates and protein to fat, but it cannot convert carbohydrates and protein—or other fat, for that matter—to the essential fatty acids. How much fat do you need in the diet? Fortunately, your need for them is small. The essential fatty acids can be obtained if only a few percent of your total calories come from fat—*particularly if they come from the unsaturated fats which are found in vegetables.*

The essential fatty acids are *linoleic acid* and *linolenic acid.* They occur widely in plant (corn, soybean) oils, and are found in animal-derived foods (meat and milk products). When linoleic and linolenic acid are furnished by the diet, the synthesis of a variety of other unsaturated fatty acids is made possible.

For example, your body must have arachidonic acid in order to produce the prostaglandins. Your body can synthesize arachidonic acid from linoleic and linolenic acids.

Essential fatty acid deficiency is rare, except in cases of severe malnutrition and in patients on long-term intravenous therapy when the administered solutions do not contain the fatty acids. However, you want your body to have a ready supply of them for immediate use. Remember, the unsaturated fats in vegetables are an excellent source of the essential fatty acids.

Ingested fats carry the lipid-soluble vitamins—vitamins A, D, E, and K. These vitamins are necessary for the optimum function of many of the systems in your body. Your body must have them if it is to continue to maintain a high-energy state and maximum youthfulness and to achieve maximum life span.

What about the fat in my typical American diet?

Having stressed the importance of obtaining the essential fatty acids, let me say that the diet of the average person in the United States contains *too much* fat. Unfortunately, most of the fat that is consumed is animal fat. Fat should provide 10-20 percent of the total dietary calories, instead of the 40-60 percent typical for many individuals. If you are one who needs to cut back on the amount of fat in your diet, be sure to continue to get the essential fatty acids.

What happens if I eat more fat than I need?

When you eat more fat than your body can use, your body stores it. We have already seen that when you eat more protein and carbohydrate than your body can use, they are converted to fat and stored. One pound of body fat contains over 3,500 calories of stored energy. If your body needs the calories, it can convert the stored fat into a usable compound and get the energy that it needs from the metabolism of that compound. In order for your body to use stored fat, the fat must first be converted (hydrolyzed) into fatty acids and glycerol. Both fatty acids and glycerol can then be changed to a compound (called acetyl coenzyme A) which can enter the citric acid cycle. The chemical processes in the citric acid cycle produce energy for the energy compound ATP.

If your body doesn't need the calories, the stored fat will remain stored. All of the calories that you ingest above your daily caloric requirement will be stored as fat. Your appestat (the part of the brain that controls food intake) will allow you to take aboard some extra calories and store them, anticipating an emergency use of them at some later time (Douglas, *Reset Your Appestat*, p. 67, QRP Books, Brandon, Miss., 1988). If you don't use the extra calories, your appestat might become permanently set at a higher level. The extra weight will stay with you.

Is storing a few extra ounces of fat all that bad?

Storing a quarter of a pound of fat each month might seem insignificant, but over a 20-year period that will amount to an extra 60 pounds of fat. People who store an excessive amount of fat get sick more often. They have more high blood pressure, heart disease, arthritis, diabetes, stomach upsets, headaches, and skin problems, more of almost any of the known diseases, than do individuals who are not overweight. They have more mood changes, more depression, and more problems with fatigue. This is not to imply that individuals who are overweight should go to any extreme to get the weight off as rapidly as possible. On the contrary, weight reduction should proceed in a gradual, programmed fashion, with the individual, all the while, eating a balanced diet.

This is made easier when fats supply 10 to 20 percent of the calories in the diet, and when the essential fatty acids are present in the fats which are ingested.

Where do proteins fit in?

The protein synthesis process (anabolism) is of primary importance. This is the mechanism by which large molecules such as hormones and antibodies are constructed from the relatively smaller molecules of amino acids.

Millions of cells are replaced in the body each second. Protein anabolism is essential for the growth and reproduction of those cells, as well as for wound healing and other tissue repair processes. Plasma proteins (prothrombin and fibrinogen) which play an important role in blood coagulation and plasma proteins (gamma globulins) which play an important role in the body's immune defense mechanism are synthesized from smaller compounds. Protein synthesis, or anabolism, is essential to the structure and function of the individual cells of the body, and thus to the structure and function of the entire body.

How does my body use amino acids?

The use of amino acids to construct proteins makes possible the formation of hormones, enzymes, tissue proteins, blood proteins, antibodies, and other compounds. All together, more than 100,000 different compounds which the body needs can be synthesized from the amino acids. Consequently, if one is to enjoy good health, it is important to have an adequate intake of amino acids—especially an adequate intake of those amino acids that the body can't synthesize, the essential amino acids.

Doesn't my body use protein as a source of energy?

If your body runs out of glucose and glycogen, it can use the body proteins as a source of energy, though this will not occur if you are eating a balanced diet. (That is a good reason in itself to avoid starvation diets and low-carbohydrate diets.)

Under normal conditions, the adult body is in a state of protein balance. That is, the rate of protein anabolism equals the rate of protein catabolism. The body is in a state of *positive* protein balance, when the buildup of body proteins exceeds the breakdown of body proteins, during growth, muscle building, and pregnancy. The body is in a state of *negative* protein balance, or "tissue wasting," when more tissue proteins are being broken down than are being replaced by protein synthesis. The causes of tissue wasting are starvation, wasting illnesses, and poor diets. Unless you are on a starvation diet, the proteins that you eat aren't usually used for energy. The proteins that you consume while on a balanced diet are used to replace your daily protein losses. They are needed for tissue repair and the other purposes which have already been discussed. Proteins—especially the essential amino acids—are necessary for these purposes, and should be properly incorporated into the diet.

Are proteins a good source of energy for my body?

Proteins aren't the ideal energy food. When they are used for energy, urea is formed, and it must be excreted by the kidneys. (Carbohydrates are different. They "burn clean," meaning that their breakdown products are carbon dioxide, which is eliminated by the lungs, and water, which can be used by the body or excreted by the kidneys.)

Of course one needs to eat enough protein to replace the daily losses, but the *quantity* of protein that one eats should be of sufficient *quality* so that one gets all of the essential amino acids.

How much protein do I need?

Since the average 150-pound man loses about 25 grams of protein a day, the recommended daily allowance for a person that size is approximately twice that, or 50 grams a day. That is a small amount, less than two ounces. Protein deficiency is a rare nutritional disorder in the United States. Even the lowest-income families consume approximately twice their average requirements of protein.

Do I have to eat meat in order to get enough protein?

No. Meats contain protein, but so do legumes (beans), breads, cereals, vegetables, oatmeal, and other foods. It would be a real challenge for you to attempt to get your daily allotment of calories by eating a variety of foods, and, at the same time, consume less than two ounces of protein. The source of the protein isn't particularly important, as long as one gets the essential amino acids. The amino acids found in plants are no different from those in meats; anyone wishing to get the essential amino acids by eating only plant proteins can do so.

If you attempted to get all of your proteins from only one plant source your diet might be deficient in one of the essential amino acids. But as long as your protein comes from a *variety* of vegetable sources, you can get all of the essential amino acids.

It is obvious that sufficient protein and the essential amino acids required for tissue repair, muscle building, and growth can be obtained from plants. Horses, cows, and other animals grow, develop, and maintain a sizable muscle mass on proteins that come from grass and grains.

It is our own initiative that is going to allow us to choose our destiny with regard to the way our bodies are going to look and function from now on (beginning today). It is our own initiative that is going to allow us to become healthier and to inhibit the aging process.

If we wait around to see how someone else fares when he takes steps to inhibit his aging process, then attempt to do likewise (to compete), we will be inhibiting our own initiative. How well we do might be controlled by how well he does. If we depend on our own initiative, we don't have to look to another individual as a "standard" by which we judge our own success in caring for our bodies. We are our own "standard" and, as such, can determine whether we are doing the best thing possible for our bodies today. We can turn our attention inward to our own health, without thought as to whether our bodies are stronger, or faster, or younger, or longer-lasting than the bodies of others. All of our efforts can be concentrated on looking, feeling, and performing better—on making our bodies last longer than they otherwise would have, had they not had our attention.

Summary

Pay attention to the basics. Perhaps before we go looking for the elixir of life, the fountain of youth, or some magic potion that will make us eternally youthful, we should first take care of the basics. We need to put that block of wood behind our trailer so that we don't send our boat down the steep ramp into the water. Here's how:

1. *Eat complex carbohydrates.*
2. *Include the essential fatty acids in your diet.*
3. *Eat three ounces of plant and/or animal protein every day. Obtain the protein from a variety of sources so that you get the essential amino acids.*
4. *Begin eating more raw fruits and vegetables.*
5. *Generate your own initiative to do these things.*

CHAPTER 5

Putting Good Nutrition to Work

Humans consume foods that come from every imaginable source. We eat varieties of every living thing that exists on, above, or beneath the land and the sea. We consume minerals, chemicals, organic and inorganic compounds.

A long process of trial and error, plus many years of vigorous scientific investigation, has helped to identify the nutrients that are ideal for human consumption. This chapter will begin a detailed discussion of those nutrients and their beneficial effects. We will also examine two completely different population groups which attain comparable levels of physical fitness even though they derive their energy from food sources that are at opposite extremes. The implication isn't that the diet of one group is just as healthy as the diet of the other group but that the human body is even more remarkable than we thought when it comes to functioning on what we feed it.

When we examine the diversity of foods on which humans can live and function, we will become aware of the incredible strength, durability, and adaptability of the human body. That should give additional credibility to the hypothesis that, given the *ideal* nutrient intake and lifestyle, the human machine can operate smoothly for a much longer time than we ever thought possible. Let's begin by taking a look at a population group that eats what most scientists today consider to be the wrong type of food.

The Masai of Tanzania, in southeast Africa, are a group of men who are unusually physically active. As boys, they spend much of their lives walking with herds of cattle. In adulthood, they walk great distances daily looking after their cattle or their property or visiting distant friends.

Years ago a group of scientists studied the Masai warriors, and concluded that they were almost free of heart and blood vessel disease

(Mann, G.V., Shaffer, R.D., and Rich, A., "Physical Fitness and Immunity to Heart Disease in Masai," *Lancet* 2:1308-1310, 1965). That was a surprising finding, considering the type of food that they eat. As it turns out, it was an incorrect conclusion (Mann, G.V., Spoerry, A., Gray, M., and Jarashow, D., "Atherosclerosis in the Masai," *American Journal of Epidemiology* 95(1):26-37, 1972). How could that have happened? Let's begin at the beginning.

Prior to the time of the first study, not everyone believed that heart and blood vessel diseases were related to the type and quantity of food that people ate. For that reason, the Masai seemed a perfect group to study in order to help settle the question. The diet of the Masai consists essentially of milk and meat. When 600 Masai were examined by clinical methods—taking the blood pressure or taking an electrocardiogram (ECG)—they showed very little evidence of heart and blood vessel disease. That prompted some scientists to interpret the results as clear evidence that heart and blood vessel diseases are unrelated to the type of food that people eat. The initial study did not include an actual examination of the blood vessels. That was unfortunate, because we now know that it is possible for a person with severe atherosclerosis (hardening of the arteries) to have a normal blood pressure and a normal ECG.

Initially, there was speculation that the high level of physical activity somehow protected the Masai from heart and blood vessel diseases. Further studies were conducted to determine whether or not that was the case. Since scientists cannot adequately measure physical activity over a long period of time, they measured one consequence of exercise—physical fitness. The results of the study were very revealing, underscoring the importance of physical activity.

To conduct the study, a group of 53 Masai males between the ages of 14 and 64 years was examined. They were asked to walk on an electrically driven treadmill which moved at the rate of approximately 3.5 miles per hour. They started walking with the treadmill surface horizontal. At the end of each minute of walking, the treadmill was raised by one degree. The volunteers walked until they were exhausted. (The speed of the treadmill remained constant, but the grade increased by one degree each minute.) The men were rewarded for taking part in the test, but the scientists who conducted the test reported that it soon became obvious that the trial was a highly competitive, attractive test of prowess for the participants. The results were astonishing.

The Masai were remarkably fit. Many of them outperformed Olympic-class athletes who were used for comparison as the control group. This observation becomes even more significant when one considers that the Masai men rarely participate in a physical activity at *maximal effort. Their persistent walking at a rate of three to five miles per hour is sufficient to maintain their high degree of fitness.* They usually walk from 10 to 20 miles *each day.* The obvious conclusion from this is that your body—your human machine—can be maintained at a high level of fitness without your having to endure the pain of daily maximal effort.

Does this high level of physical fitness protect the Masai against heart and blood vessel disease?

No, the Masai survive well into adulthood *in spite of* the atherosclerosis that develops as a result of their diet of milk and meat.

That Masai do have atherosclerosis was confirmed when the hearts and blood vessels of 50 men, who had died suddenly of accidents or other causes, were examined. The aorta, the largest artery in the body, showed extensive atherosclerosis, with fat infiltration into the wall of the vessel. The coronary arteries, which supply blood to the heart, showed wall thickening which equaled or surpassed that of elderly American men. Why then does atherosclerosis not cause Masai men to die at an early age? Apparently their high level of physical activity over a lifetime causes their blood vessels to enlarge enough with age to partially compensate for the atherosclerosis. (Note: In neither of the studies was there mention of men who were beyond their 60s. Apparently even very high levels of physical activity will not compensate totally for a diet which produces atherosclerosis.)

High blood pressure is unusual among the Masai, and the blood pressure does not increase with age as it does in the Western world. Their high level of physical activity is also probably responsible for this.

The Masai are not fat, despite their diet—again, a reflection of the large number of calories they burn each day by walking. The adult Masai men are about the same height as American men, but they are about 10 kilograms (approximately 22 pounds) lighter. Imagine what a devastating effect a diet of nothing but milk and meat would have on an inactive, overweight person. His entire system of blood vessels would be wrecked in short order.

What about the other side of the coin? How physically active could an individual be if his diet consisted almost exclusively of carbohydrates? Would he have enough energy to get through the day? Could he develop his muscles? Would he have endurance? We gained some insight into those questions when we examined the diets of people who compete in marathons and triathlons. What about population groups who eat a high carbohydrate diet routinely over a lifetime? Let's take a brief look at such a group.

In Mexico, a group of peoples known as the Taracahitian includes the Tarahumaras of southern Sonora and Chihuahua. The diet of the Tarahumaras, which consists mainly of carbohydrates, is almost exactly the opposite of the Masai diet, which comprises primarily protein and fat.

Pritikin drew attention to the Tarahumaras in 1979. They eat corn, beans, squash, native plants, and fruits. Infrequently—perhaps once a month—they consume some animal protein. Approximately 80 percent of their calories comes from carbohydrates, with the remaining calories coming from fat and protein. The diet of the Tarahumaras probably isn't ideal. They have high infant and childhood mortality rates. (However, it's likely that some of the infant and childhood deaths are due to the lack of medical care and to diseases, not to malnutrition.) Even so, the Tarahumaras, like the Masai, are capable of prolonged physical activity.

The Tarahumaras assume a slow trot when they play their kickball game. The game might last a couple of days, during which time men playing the game cover distances of 50 miles or more. Women play too, but because of their family responsibilities they run shorter distances. Since the Tarahumaras are in such good physical condition, it isn't difficult for them to trot for two days or to walk long distances carrying heavy packs.

According to Pritikin, physicians who have examined these people find them free of cardiovascular disease, diabetes, and obesity. This is not surprising, since high-fat diets and high blood-lipid (fat) levels promote the development of cardiovascular disease, whereas high-carbohydrate/low-fat diets are associated with a low incidence of cardiovascular disease. Physical activity also influences the rate of development of cardiovascular disease as well as other degenerative diseases. High levels of aerobic exercise lower the blood pressure, decrease the heart rate, have a positive effect on glucose tolerance, reduce the level of the harmful low-density lipoproteins in the blood, raise the level of the beneficial high-density lipoproteins in the blood, help reduce mental stress, and increase life expectancy (Douglas, 1988, and Paffenbarger, et al, 1986).

There is no need to worry about having a lack of strength and endurance on a high-carbohydrate, low-fat diet. The Tarahumaras lack neither strength nor endurance. Also, we have already seen that the well-trained athlete can complete a grueling triathlon which may take 14 or more hours. All of these extraordinary feats can be accomplished on high-carbohydrate, low-fat diets.

What good will diet and exercise do if you already have heart disease?

Is heart disease reversible? Yes! Now there is some exciting new evidence to indicate that lifestyle changes can help *reverse* heart disease. Dr. Dean Ornish, at the American Heart Association's 61st Scientific Sessions (1988), reported on two groups of patients with blocked coronary arteries. (Many were serious enough to require bypass surgery.) The first group of patients underwent comprehensive lifestyle changes. They learned to manage stress; they received group counseling; they quit smoking; they exercised; and they ate a vegetarian diet which contained only 10 percent fat. The second group of patients exercised; they quit smoking; and they ate a standard low-fat diet which contained 30 percent fat. The two groups were compared a year later. The artery blockage dropped significantly in the first group, whose diet contained 10 percent fat, while it increased in the others. According to Dr. Ornish, the best results were seen in patients who were older and had greater blockage initially. Here then, is scientific evidence that changes in lifestyle can begin to reverse coronary blockages. Without evidence such as this, one might make wrong conclusions regarding diets.

A cursory examination of the diets of the Masai and the Tarahumaras might seem to indicate that one has two choices with regard to diet, and that either choice is acceptable as long as one gets enough exercise. One might also conclude that a compromise such as the American diet of 40-50 percent fat and protein, is the best solution. *Wrong.* There is just too much scientific evidence against such a conclusion. The fact that the peoples in the two cultures are capable of extraordinary physical feats on diets that are strikingly different doesn't prove that the two diets are equally acceptable, only that the human body is capable of extraordinary adaptation.

Can I eat whatever I want as long as I get enough exercise?

Not if you want to maintain optimum health. We have to remember that, though the Masai perform well on their diet, they do have severe atherosclerosis. Besides, how many among us have the *time* to walk 10 to 20 miles a day, every day, in order to live a little longer while we eat foods that produce atherosclerosis? Wouldn't it be better to live a lot longer by engaging in moderate exercise *and* by eating foods that don't produce atherosclerosis?

Perhaps you have surmised from the preceding information that even though the human body is capable of adapting to a multitude of different foods, one dietary combination is preferred over all the others. I believe the human body is designed so that it will function best on a diet in which:

Carbohydrates provide 70-75 percent of the calories;
Proteins provide 15 percent of the calories;
Fats provide the remaining 10-15 percent of the calories.

But will I feel better?

It is my firm belief that if you adopt this nutrition combination as a way of life, you will notice a difference within 24 hours, and that within 30 days you will feel like a new person. Feeding your body in this fashion will do more to inhibit the aging process than any other way of eating and will also increase your life expectancy.

A diet with this combination of foods is easy to achieve. (Basically, if you concentrate on eating fruits, vegetables, and grains, you stand a very good chance of getting sufficient protein and fat in the process without even having to worry about it, but more about that later.) A diet with this combination of foods promotes good health, is economical, and is so palatable that once individuals become accustomed to it, they look forward to trying different food combinations, and there is limitless opportunity for experimentation with food combinations. Further, they feel so good that they wouldn't consider returning to the old all-American (40 per cent fat) diet, even if someone could convince them that it too is healthy.

A high-carbohydrate, low-fat, low-protein diet will go a long way toward reducing the incidence of atherosclerosis, obesity, high blood pressure, diabetes, degenerative diseases, fatigue, and many other conditions with which people must contend. A diet such as this typically produces a dramatic increase in the energy level of individuals. Many individuals who have switched to this type of diet have wondered why they spent so many years as a "couch potato."

PLEASE NOTE: *This type of diet is recommended for people who consider themselves healthy. If you are on prescription drugs or if you are undergoing medical treatment, consult your physician before making major changes in your diet or lifestyle. Individuals put themselves at risk when they attempt to solve medical problems without the advice of trained medical professionals.*

Isn't this going to be a chore to eat right? No. You are about to experience a very pleasant phenomenon. As you switch to this new combination of foods, your physical strength and stamina will increase. These foods will provide you with additional energy and endurance just as surely as grains and vegetables provide energy and endurance to the thoroughbred racehorse. That will be a pleasant enough experience within itself, but I am referring to an additional experience—an additional bonus, if you will—to be gained by pursuing this new lifestyle. I believe you will become "addicted" to doing good things for your body.

When you become positively addicted to one thing and gain strength in that area as a result of the addiction, *that strength will spill over into other areas.* This process and the reasons for it have been thoroughly analyzed (Glasser, W., *Positive Addiction*, Harper and Row, New York, 1976). That spillover of strength is going to affect almost every facet of your life. Doing one beneficial thing for your body will automatically provide the stimulus for doing something else beneficial for it. This attitude applies to our present concern: the prevention of premature aging.

What can a positive addiction do for me?

The positive addiction of supplying your body with the proper nutrients, as well as following other guidelines provided in this book, will essentially eliminate the feeling that it is less painful to give up than to keep moving toward a goal—whether it's a goal of preventing premature aging or any other goal toward which you might be moving. Positive addictions will help you to become mentally and physically stronger. The more strength you have, the more likely you are to work out a problem when it confronts you and to try new approaches to problems as they occur. You will evolve from a state of less-than-optimal strength (with limited options to solve problems) to a state of maximum strength with the attendant energy to exercise new options for problem-solving.

You will notice this effect regardless of your age, sex, or occupation. That boring or mundane part of your job or life will be less noticeable because of your increased mental and physical strength, and you will be able to take care of that extra chore, or to exercise more, almost without giving it a thought.

You will have renewed enthusiasm for charging on toward the goal of living out your 110-year life span. With new positive addictions, giving up on the goal will not even be a consideration.

Increased mental and physical strength will have another beneficial effect. The tendency to move in the opposite direction—that is, toward negative addictions—will be eliminated. As you develop positive addictions, you won't be inclined to putter about during the day and then plop down in front of the TV at night with a beer and a plate of high-fat food. We can't develop positive addictions and negative addictions at the same time. The actions are just as incompatible as trying to run a 100-yard dash while smoking a cigarette. The two are just mutually exclusive.

When individuals develop positive addictions, many chronic, nagging symptoms disappear. Strengthened individuals experience fewer headaches, backaches, muscle pains, or other aches and pains. They frequently experience less depression, anxiety, and tenseness, and feel less apprehension about dealing with people or situations.

Proper feeding of the body bathes each cell of the body with a fluid, known as extracellular fluid, which contains the optimum combination of water, food, vitamins, and minerals to prolong the health and life of the cell. Let us explore briefly the process of maintaining the best possible combination of ingredients in that extracellular fluid.

Much of the body—about 60 percent—is fluid. The fluid inside the cells of the body is known as the *intracellular* fluid. The fluid outside the cells, which bathes the cells, is known as the *extracellular* fluid. Within the extracellular fluid are the dissolved constituents used by the cells for the maintenance of life.

This extracellular fluid is always in motion and is constantly mixing throughout the body. For that reason, all of the cells of the body live in the same environment. The fluid surrounding one cell is essentially identical to the fluid surrounding another. Because of that, the extracellular fluid has been called the internal environment of the body.

As long as the extracellular fluid contains oxygen, carbohydrates (particularly glucose), amino acids, fatty acids, vitamins, and minerals, the cells of the body are capable of living, growing, reproducing, and repairing themselves. Oxygen and nutrients are constantly being added to the extracellular fluid; carbon dioxide and waste products are constantly being removed from it. The very best thing that individuals can do for the cells of their body is to add a good supply of quality nutrients to the extracellular fluid.

How are quality nutrients added to the extracellular fluid?

When the heart beats, it pumps blood around and around the circulatory system. The blood flows from the heart into the arteries and then into the capillaries. From the capillaries it flows into the veins and from the veins back into the heart. The capillaries are porous so that fluid can diffuse back and forth between the blood and the spaces around the cells. As the blood passes through the capillaries, fluid carrying oxygen and nutrients flows out of the capillaries and around the cells. At the same time fluid from around the cells (which is carrying carbon dioxide and waste products) flows back into the capillaries. This exchange of fluid takes place constantly, 24 hours a day, whether you are awake or asleep, active or inactive.

Maintaining a good flow of blood through the capillaries is extremely important to the continued good health of the cells of the body. There are so many capillaries in the body that practically no cell is located more than 50 microns (about 1/500th of an inch) from a capillary. This allows for the extremely rapid movement of any substance from the blood to the cells, or from the cells back to the blood.

When a person is at rest, all of the blood in the circulatory system goes around the entire circuit an average of once each minute. It might go around as many as five times a minute during vigorous exercise. When blood flows through the lungs, it picks up oxygen and gives up carbon dioxide. When it flows through the digestive tract, it picks up water, vitamins, minerals, carbohydrates, fatty acids, and amino acids which can be transported to the extracellular fluid. The blood also picks up hormones from the glands of the body, as well as compounds which the liver has produced. The hormones can influence the function of the cells, and the cells can use the compounds which the liver has produced. These can pass from the blood through the walls of the capillaries into the extracellular fluid.

The kidneys filter blood as it flows through them. The beneficial substances, including water, if it is needed, are kept by the body, and the waste products are excreted. This makes the kidneys powerful, automatic regulators both of the volume of the extracellular fluid and the materials which it contains.

An encompassing statement has been made regarding the optimum combination of foods for sustaining long-term health. The proper percentages of carbohydrates, fat, and protein in the diet are important, but the diet should contain a sufficient variety of foods so that the necessary vitamins, minerals, and trace elements are consumed. The proper intake of nutrients, together with the kidney's ability to excrete or keep that which the body needs, will ensure that each cell of the body is bathed with the ideal extracellular fluid.

Summary

Selecting the proper foods need not be a cumbersome, complicated process. You don't have to have a master's degree in nutrition or surround yourself with charts and tables in order to select the proper foods. That will become apparent when the food sources of various nutrients are discussed in the next chapter. For the time being, we can say it in 20 words or less: "Eat the proper percentages of carbohydrates, fat, and protein, and, in the process, eat a large variety of foods."

To help prevent premature aging:

1. *Don't eat a diet similar to that of the Masai (only meat and milk).*
2. *Do eat a diet with the proper percentages of nutrients.*
3. *Eat a diet compatible with stabilizing, or reversing coronary atherosclerosis.*
4. *See that the cells of your body are bathed with the ideal extracellular fluid.*
5. *Develop a positive addiction for caring for your body.*

CHAPTER 6

Vitamins, Minerals
and Trace Elements
for Inhibiting Aging

Almost everyone knows that aging is not a disease. Most also agree that being happy and deriving pleasure from life contribute as much to longevity as do pills and other medicines. We cannot, at the present time, stop the aging clock, but we have the potential for living much longer than we do now. We can extend our current life expectancy by 40 years or more. In that regard, good nutrition is vitally important because nutrient intake influences what goes on in each cell of the body. The following information is designed to provide information to help you with a program of nutrition. Let us consider some essential nutrients.

A balanced diet should contain enough water-soluble vitamins for an ample supply to the extracellular fluid. The water-soluble vitamins, their functions, and the foods which contain them are discussed below.

Water-soluble Vitamins.
A vitamin to help your metabolism. Vitamin B1 (thiamine) functions in the human metabolic system. Because thiamine deficiency interferes with the utilization of pyruvic acid, thiamine is essential for the final metabolism of carbohydrates. Thiamine is found in meats, whole grains, and legumes.

Two vitamins for your energy system. Vitamin B2 (riboflavin) usually combines with phosphoric acid and proteins to form substances called flavoproteins. The flavoproteins act as hydrogen carriers in some of the energy systems of the body. This allows for the efficient formation of the energy compound ATP. Severe riboflavin deficiency in the human is rare, but a mild deficiency is common. Symptoms include cracking of the skin at the corners of the mouth, burning sensations of the skin, digestive disturbances, headaches, and depression. Though symptoms of riboflavin deficiency alone are mild, the condition usually occurs in association with a deficiency of other substances such as thiamine or niacin. Riboflavin is found in legumes, meats, dairy products, and grains.

Niacin functions in the energy system of the body. When a deficiency exists, energy cannot be delivered at normal rates from the foods to the elements in the cells which use the energy. Niacin deficiency depresses *all* of the functions of the body. It causes scaliness of the skin, inflammation of the mucous membranes of the mouth, muscle weakness, poor glandular secretion, and, in severe cases, tissue death. Niacin deficiency generally seems to make tissue repair difficult. Niacin is found in dried beans, soybeans, asparagus, collards, corn, barley, wheat, cold-water fish, beef, and chicken.

A vitamin to assist with protein metabolism. Vitamin B6 (pyridoxine) functions in many chemical reactions in the body relating to amino acid and protein metabolism. It is important for the conversion of amino acids into substances which the cells can use. Pure pyridoxine deficiency occurs infrequently; it is usually in association with a deficiency of other vitamins. (An insufficient amount of pyridoxine in lower animals results in a slowed growth rate and evidence of mental deterioration.) Pyridoxine is found in vegetables, whole grain cereals, milk, and meats.

A vitamin to assist with carbohydrate and fat metabolism. Pantothenic acid has many important metabolic roles in the body. It is incorporated into a substance called co-enzyme A, which is essential for the conversion of pyruvic acid and for the degradation of fatty acid molecules. It follows that a lack of pantothenic acid leads to depressed metabolism of both carbohydrates and fats. While a frank deficiency of pantothenic acid isn't likely, an ample quantity in the body means that the metabolism of carbohydrates and fats can proceed in the most efficient fashion possible. Fruits, vegetables, cereals, milk, and meats contain pantothenic acid.

Two vitamins that promote growth and repair. Folic acid is an important growth promoter, probably more so than vitamin B12. Millions of cells in the body must be replaced *daily*. Folic acid is necessary for the reproduction of the genes in the cells, and a good supply of folic acid in the diet will assure that quick, efficient cell reproduction can take place to replace those cells which have died or which have been destroyed. Folic acid, like vitamin B12, is important for the maturation of the red blood cells; a deficiency of either of these vitamins may cause anemia. Although both folic acid and vitamin B12 are important to the growth of cells, they function differently and thus are not interchangeable. One cannot be substituted for the other. Cereals, vegetables, fruits, and meats contain folic acid.

Vitamin B12 (cyanocobalamin), like folic acid, is a promoter of growth. It is important in the formation of a substance known as thymine, a lack of which limits the formation of genes, thereby reducing the rate at which the cells of the body can divide. An ample supply of vitamin B12 in the body means that cell reproduction can more easily take place at a sufficient rate to replace those which have been lost. If vitamin B12 is poorly absorbed from the intestine, an anemia (pernicious anemia) develops because red blood cells can't be produced fast enough. Vitamin B12 also helps keep the large nerve fibers healthy. Vitamin B12 deficiency causes a demyelination (loss of covering) of some of the large nerve fibers of the spinal cord.

NOTE: Since vitamin B12 is one of the water-soluble vitamins, it cannot be stored in the body for prolonged periods of time. Also, since it is found in meats and dairy products and does not occur in plants, vegan vegetarians might want to consult their physician about taking vitamin B12 supplements. Some foods are "fortified" with vitamin B12, but not always to the extent that they can supply the recommended daily allowance.

Vitamins for efficient metabolism, neutral fat reduction in the liver, and rapid tissue repair. *Biotin* is needed by the body for efficient carbohydrate metabolism and also probably for the formation of fatty acids and for protein metabolism. A good supply of biotin in the diet can help prevent lassitude, gastrointestinal symptoms, and some mild dermatitis symptoms. Legumes, vegetables, and meats contain this vitamin.

Choline is utilized by the liver to produce lecithin, which reduces the amount of neutral fat in the liver. Choline is also a source of substances (methyl radicals) used by the body for the detoxification of many toxic compounds. Choline is necessary for the production of a substance known as acetylcholine, a compound essential for the transmission of nerve impulses in the body. Choline is present in grains, legumes, and liver.

Vitamin C (ascorbic acid) has probably received more attention than any of the other water-soluble vitamins. Some of the claims which have been made for its action are justified; other have not been experimentally verified.

Ascorbic acid is a compound which probably acts in the metabolic process to reversibly exchange electrons with different energy systems. Its main function seems to be to maintain the structural substances such as collagen and the intercellular cement between the cells of the body. A deficiency of ascorbic acid slows the rate of wound healing and of bone growth and repair and can cause the blood vessel walls to become more fragile. If this happens, capillaries in the body are likely to rupture, with the resulting formation of bluish-purple spots over the skin.

A complete absence of ascorbic acid can become almost lethal within about two months. Prolonged, severe ascorbic acid deficiency causes scurvy. Symptoms are bleeding gums, loose teeth, fragmentation of muscle cells, fragile blood vessels, perhaps a high fever, and finally a stroke.

An adequate intake of ascorbic acid results in better maintenance of collagen in the skin (and in other parts of the body), healthier blood vessels, and a boost to the overall metabolic processes.

People who eat citrus fruits and raw vegetables, such as tomatoes, get a good supply of ascorbic acid.

Why is it important for me to have a constant infusion of water-soluble vitamins?

Since the water-soluble vitamins stay in the body for only a short period of time, it is important to provide a constant infusion of them. This is especially true of the B-vitamins. Clinical symptoms of a B-vitamin deficiency can appear within a few days, and, as we have seen, a deficiency of vitamin C can become dangerous within a matter of weeks.

You can have a constant infusion of the water-soluble vitamins by eating the foods which contain them on a continuing basis. You cannot get this result by taking large doses of these vitamins and then expecting the body to store them for later release. The body doesn't store the water-soluble vitamins; they are threshold substances for excretion by the kidneys. When large doses are taken, the excess will be excreted almost immediately by the kidneys. Your body is more likely to remain highly energized and healthy if your water-soluble vitamins are obtained from foods rather than from vitamin supplements.

When you get a constant infusion of the water-soluble vitamins from food sources, you are getting the complex carbohydrate, fiber, and minerals from the foods along with the vitamins. No matter what food supplements you may be taking, you can probably improve your nutritional status, beginning today, by regularly eating foods which contain the water-soluble vitamins. It isn't necessary to eat different foods each day, but over a period of a month it is probably best to eat as much of a variety of foods as possible. That should keep a steady, varied supply of vitamins, minerals, and trace elements pouring into your system.

Your body also needs the fat-soluble vitamins. Let's examine the reasons.

Fat-Soluble Vitamins.

A vitamin that prevents night blindness and promotes skin health. *Vitamin A* is necessary for the formation of retinal pigments and thus serves to prevent night blindness. This vitamin is also important for normal growth and reproduction of most cells of the body, particularly skin cells. Vitamin A deficiency will cause scaliness of the skin, and often the damaged skin areas become infected. For that reason, vitamin A has been called the ''anti-infection'' vitamin. A deficiency will cause kidney stones, probably as a result of infection of the space—the renal pelvic—in the kidney which collects urine.

Vitamin A occurs in milk and milk products. It occurs as provitamins in vegetables such as broccoli, carrots, collards, mustard greens, sweet potatoes, and spinach. These provitamins have chemical structures which are similar to vitamin A and can be changed into vitamin A in the human body.

Too much vitamin A is harmful, but when you have the optimum supply in your body, your vision will be enhanced and so will the growth and reproduction of your cells. I have heard it said that eating green vegetables makes the skin look healthy. It does, and vitamin A is the reason.

A vitamin for healthy bones. *Vitamin D* is found in fish-liver oils, dairy products, and eggs, but the body can get an adequate supply of this vitamin from other sources. The body can produce vitamin D when sunlight (ultraviolet irradiation) strikes the skin and converts a substance there (7-dehydrocholesterol) into a compound referred to as the natural vitamin D (vitamin D3). A synthetic vitamin D compound, calciferol, is used in vitamin-D therapy.

The vitamin D in the body increases the absorption of calcium and phosphate from the digestive tract. These substances are essential for bone growth and repair. Control of the level of calcium in the body is also essential to good health.

A vitamin to increase the sex drive? *Vitamin E* promotes normal growth. Many different compounds exhibit vitamin E activity. When scientists refer to "vitamin E," they are usually referring to the compound alpha-tocopherol.

Experiments have shown that a lack of vitamin E can cause a degeneration of the germinal tissue in the testes of lower animals. Since it seems necessary for healthy testicular function, vitamin E is sometimes referred to as the anti-sterility vitamin. Both men and women have claimed that it increases their sex drive, but this is evidence of an anecdotal nature, not the result of well-designed scientific studies. At any rate, vitamin E has been associated with a healthy reproductive system.

Since vitamin E promotes the normal growth of the cells of the body, it affects every system of the body. It is said to enhance the immune system and stimulate antibody production, thereby increasing the resistance to bacterial infection. Vitamin E inhibits the formation of free radicals. (Free radicals form during the process of normal metabolism. They flail about inside and outside the cells of the body causing some destruction and thus contributing to the aging process.) For these reasons, vitamin E is sometimes thought of as a youth-promoting vitamin.

Vitamin E is found in green leafy vegetables, seeds, and shortenings.

Protection from hemorrhage in the form of a vitamin. *Vitamin K* activity is exhibited in several different natural and synthetic compounds. Vitamin K is necessary for the the liver's formation of substances (prothrombin and factor VII) which are important in blood clotting.

In humans, vitamin K is synthesized by bacteria in the large intestine (colon). Because of this, a dietary source of this vitamin is usually not necessary. However, if the bacteria of the colon are destroyed by large doses of antibiotics, vitamin K deficiency can rapidly develop.

Vitamin K is found in green leafy vegetables, fruits, meats, and some cereals. (As a matter of fact, your body can produce vitamin D, and *all* of the other fat-soluble vitamins are found in green leafy vegetables.)

Minerals.

In order to function efficiently, your body also needs a variety of minerals. A deficiency of one or more of the required minerals can have devastating effects on your daily performance and on the aging process.

We sometimes classify the minerals that we need as either "primary" minerals or "trace" minerals. This is an artificial classification. A trace mineral may be just as important as one of the primary minerals, even though the body might require a smaller quantity of it.

The minerals that the body needs are found in the leaf, fruit, seed, and root systems of plants, in the waters of rivers and lakes, and in animal-derived foods. (The animals from which the foods are derived get their minerals from water, vegetable, and grain sources.)

With minerals, as with vitamins, more isn't necessarily better. If you overload your body with an essential mineral, the effects might be just as detrimental as a deficiency of that mineral. Consequently, mineral supplements probably shouldn't be considered unless a mineral deficiency has been demonstrated. *I am* in favor of increasing the intake of vitamins and minerals, *provided it is done in the fashion described in Chapter Seven.*

Let's examine briefly the role of the "major" minerals and the "trace" elements.

A mineral for bone growth and repair. Calcium, which is present in the body primarily as calcium phosphate in the bones, is essential for bone growth and repair as well as for proper nerve conduction and muscle contraction. Many physicians recommend that the calcium intake in women be increased from 1,000 to 1,200 milligrams per day before age 35 and to 1,500 to 2,000 milligrams per day beginning at about 35 years of age. The reasons for this will be given during the discussion of ways to prevent premature aging of the skeletal system.

Calcium is present in dark green vegetables, legumes, and milk products). If you attempt to get all of your calcium from high-protein foods, the amount of calcium absorbed may actually be decreased. You can get an extra 300 milligrams of calcium each day by eating (for example) 1 cup of collard greens, 1 cup of plain yogurt, or 1 1/2 ounces of Cheddar cheese.

Consult your physician before taking calcium supplements. If you do take calcium supplements, the best form is probably calcium carbonate, the compound found in antacid tablets.

Two elements needed for body-water balance and nerve conduction. *Sodium* maintains the electrical potentials across nerves and muscles. This makes it possible for the nerves to conduct impulses and for the muscles to contract. Sodium is the major cation (positively charged ion) in the extracellular fluid and is important in body-water balance. Most American diets contain too much sodium.

Chlorine. The chloride ion is the major anion (negatively charged ion) in the extracellular fluid and, in association with sodium, is important in both body-water balance and acid-base balance. Most American diets contain too much chlorine in the form of sodium chloride, or table salt.

A mineral that offers protection from stroke? *Potassium* is essential for normal nerve and muscle function and for acid-base balance. There is also evidence that a high intake of dietary potassium provides protection against death from stroke. The findings are based on a 12-year study of 859 men and women between the ages of 50 and 79 (quoted from the *Journal of the Dental Assistant* 56(6):12, 1987).

The relationship between dietary potassium and stroke mortality was still strong even after accounting for other risk factors, such as high blood pressure, cigarette smoking, age, sex, blood-cholesterol level, and fasting blood-glucose level.

The results of the above study indicate that one extra serving of fresh fruits or vegetables a day may decrease the risk of stroke by as much as 40 percent.

Magnesium is required for many enzymatic reactions which take place on the inside of the cells of the body, particularly those relating to carbohydrate metabolism.

Whole grains and green leafy vegetables contain magnesium.

Energy from a mineral? *Phosphorus* is the major anion (negatively charged particle) in the fluid inside the cells. It functions with a number of enzyme systems and other compounds necessary for the operation of the metabolic process. Phosphates make up a part of the energy compound ATP (adenosine triphosphate) and phosphates are probably the most important minerals for cellular activity.

Grains, milk products, poultry, and meats contain phosphorus.

A mineral that forms hemoglobin. Iron must be present so that the body can form hemoglobin, the compound inside the red blood cells that transports oxygen. Certain enzymes (oxidative enzymes) inside the other cells of the body also contain iron. Without iron for the transport of oxygen to the tissues and for the maintenance of the oxidative enzyme systems, life would cease within a matter of seconds. Iron deficiency can cause fatigue, irritability, lethargy, and headaches.

Iron deficiency may be a problem in children and in women in the child-bearing years, but it usually isn't in others. It's estimated that women between the ages of 12 and 50 get only about two-thirds of the amount of iron that they need. Women in this age group need about 18 milligrams of iron a day.

The iron needs of men and postmenopausal women are about half that of younger women. Only one in 500 adult males has iron deficiency anemia (Cook, et al, *Blood* 68:726-731, 1986). If adult men and postmenopausal women are eating a balanced diet, are not anemic, and haven't been told by a physician to take iron supplements, it probably isn't necessary.

Iron supplements ads are so effective that 10 to 20 percent of adults are taking unnecessary pills. This is not in their best interest, as too much iron can be harmful. One study (Stevens, R., *New England Journal of Medicine,* Oct. 10, 1988) has shown that too much iron in the body can increase the long-term risk of all types of cancer. This study showed that men with high levels of iron in their bodies have a 40 percent higher cancer risk. A smaller cancer risk was found in women with high levels of iron in their bodies.

Excess iron can cause another disorder. Iron overdose in susceptible individuals may cause a disease that can damage the heart, liver, and pancreas due to an accumulation of the mineral in these organs. The disease is known as *hemochromatosis.*

Iron supplements recommended by physicians for women in the child-bearing years probably don't raise the iron level in the body enough to create a cancer risk. Also, iron-fortified foods are probaby still good for growing children. Their needs for iron are different from the needs of adults.

A balanced diet is the best source of iron. You can get iron from green leafy vegetables, legumes, whole grains, and lean meats.

A mineral for the immune system, for the maintenance of potency, for an enzyme system, and for digestion. Zinc is a part of the enzyme carbonic anhydrase. This enzyme is present in high concentration in the red blood cells. There it functions to rapidly transport carbon dioxide from the tissues of the body to the lungs, where the carbon dioxide is released. Carbonic anhydrase is also present in the gastrointestinal tract, the kidneys, the various glands of the body, and the pancreas and is vital to their function.

Zinc is a component of an enzyme that is necessary for the digestion of proteins in the gastrointestinal tract. This mineral is also vital to the health of the immune system. Claims have been made that zinc is a crucial factor in the male sexual system, in that it helps maintain potency and make strong, healthy sperm.

Zinc deficiency can cause growth retardation, skin rashes, immune deficiency, diarrhea, night blindness, impaired glucose tolerance, and diminished wound healing, and may possibly alter taste sensations (Wilkins and Levinsky, 1983).

This doesn't mean that everyone should start taking zinc supplements. Too much zinc might actually make the immune system and other body systems operate at something less than peak efficiency. I am convinced that the safest course to follow is to get zinc from foods which contain it.

The daily requirement of zinc is unknown. This versatile mineral is present in the root system and leafy parts of plants which have been grown in soil that contains zinc, and can also be found in foods derived from animals which eat those plants. Seafoods are also a good source.

Other minerals and trace elements which promote good health.

Fluorine is found in seafood and is usually added to municipal drinking water. It doesn't seem to be necessary for metabolism in the body, but small quantities of it in the body during the time when teeth are developing protect against tooth decay.

Iodine, the best known of the trace elements, is essential for the formation of thyroxin, a hormone produced by the thyroid gland. Thyroxin helps to maintain the normal metabolic rates of all of the cells of the body.

Goiters form when the body doesn't have enough iodine. Iodine is present in some foods, but humans get it primarily from iodized salt.

Manganese is essential for the activation of one of the major enzymes (arginase) necessary for the formation of urea. If arginase can't be activated, ammonium compounds in the body can't be converted into urea. As a result, ammonium will accumulate in the body fluids, causing toxicity. Manganese activates many of the metabolic enzymes in the body, including at least one necessary for the breakdown of glycogen. Manganese deficiency in the diet of animals causes atrophy of the testicles. One report *(Journal of Nutrition* 118:764-773, 1988) indicates that many people may not be getting enough manganese in their diet. According to the report, the lower end of the recommended range of manganese (2.5 to 5.0 milligrams) may be too low for men. It was suggested that a range of 3.5 to 7.0 milligrams/day would be more appropriate and would perhaps prevent men from being in negative manganese balance.

Tea, rice, and fruits contain manganese.

Copper deficiency is rare, though it has occurred in infants receiving only a milk diet. These infants have small red blood cells. Copper deficiency inhibits the ability of the bone marrow to synthesize hemoglobin. It also inhibits the absorption of iron from the gastrointestinal tract and decreases the quantities of iron-containing enzymes in the cells of the body. Copper deficiency might affect the immune system and likely affects the ability of the thyroid gland to secrete its hormones. The daily requirement of copper is unknown.

An adequate level of copper in the body can be maintained by the occasional inclusion of foods such as lobster, oysters, and fortified bran in the diet.

Cobalt is needed by the human body but not in the ionic form, or "pure" cobalt. The need is for a preformed cobalt compound, vitamin B12. Cobalt is an essential part of vitamin B12, which appears to have a role in the formation of the structural component of the red blood cell. It apparently isn't involved in the formation of the hemoglobin inside the red blood cells. Too much cobalt in the diet causes the formation of an increased number of red blood cells which have a reduced hemoglobin content—another of the many reasons to avoid overloading your body with "megadoses" of vitamins, minerals, and trace elements.

The preformed cobalt compound, vitamin B12, is found in meats and dairy products.

Selenium is an important trace element, though not all of its roles have been elucidated. Claims have been made that the proper levels of selenium enhance antibody formation and reduce the incidence of certain cancers in animals, and that a deficiency can make the immune system less active. Selenium is present in semen and is believed by some to be necessary for optimum sexual function. Selenium deficiency may result in muscle tenderness, and it might make the red blood cells more fragile. There are several food sources of selenium, including grains, bran, wheat germ, broccoli, and clams.

Chromium potentiates the action of insulin. A deficiency is associated with impaired glucose tolerance and elevated serum cholesterol levels. Chromium is present in beer, beef, black pepper, and some vegetables.

Molybdenum is a component of several enzymes in the body, such as xanthine oxidase, a flavoprotein. Flavoproteins catalyze a wide variety of (oxidation-reduction) reactions in the body. Molybdenum is also a component of aldehyde oxidase, a liver enzyme.

Cereals, buckwheat, and tomato sauce contain molybdenum.

Summary

The 15 trace elements believed to be essential to nonhuman animals are arsenic, chromium, cobalt, copper, fluorine, iodine, iron, manganese, molybdenum, nickel, selenium, silicon, tin, vanadium, and zinc.

The elements considered essential to humans were discussed above. Those which, thus far, are *not* considered essential in humans are arsenic, fluorine, nickel, silicon, tin, and vanadium. (Fluorine, although not considered essential, was included in the discussion above because of its effect on the prevention of tooth decay.)

Get into the thick of the action: Begin preventing the premature aging of your body today by eating the foods which contain vitamins, minerals, and trace elements.

VITAMIN AND MINERAL SOURCES

Water-soluble Vitamins

Vitamin B1 (thiamine) - Beef, ham, pork chops, cooked dry beans, legumes, whole grains, whole wheat flour

Vitamin B2 (riboflavin) - Legumes, kidney beans, black-eyed peas, meats, dairy products, grains, fortified cereals

Niacin - Dried beans, soybeans, asparagus, collards, corn, barley, wheat, cold-water fish, beef, chicken

Vitamin B6 (pyridoxine) - Whole grain cereals, milk, meats, bananas, cooked dry beans, spinach

Pantothenic Acid - Fruits, cereals, milk, meats, eggs, mushrooms

Folic Acid - Cereals, fruits, meats, turnip greens, mustard, orange juice, cooked dry beans, asparagus

Vitamin B12 (cyanocobalamin) - Beef, lamb, fish, dairy products, yeast extracts

Biotin - Peas, beans, soybeans, oatmeal, clams, milk, meats

Choline - Grains, peas, beans, liver

Vitamin C (ascorbic acid) - Oranges, lemons, limes, grapefruit, kiwi fruit, broccoli, green peppers, tomatoes

Fat-soluble Vitamins

Vitamin A - Milk, dairy products, broccoli, carrots, collards, mustard greens, sweet potatoes, spinach

Vitamin D - Fish-liver oils, fresh water fish, milk products, eggs, sunlight

Vitamin E - Spinach, turnip greens, green leafy vegetables, seeds, nuts, vegetable oils and shortenings

Vitamin K - Turnip greens, lettuce, cabbage, broccoli, green leafy vegetables, fruits, meats, some cereals

Minerals

Calcium - Turnips, mustard greens, milk products, peas, beans

Sodium - Table salt, meat, seafood

Chlorine - Table salt, meat, seafood

Potassium - Orange juice, baked potato, kidney beans, avocados, bananas, salmon, tomataoes, fruits, vegetables

Magnesium - Turnips, beat greens, dry beans, avocados, bananas, whole grains, green leafy vegetables

Phosphorus - Grains, milk products, poultry, fish, meats, dry beans

Iron - Green leafy vegetables, dry beans, dry peas, whole grains, fortified cereals, blackstrap molasses, lean meats

Zinc - Seafoods, wheat, beans, dairy products, leafy parts of vegetables grown in soil that contains zinc, foods derived from animals which eat those plants

Fluorine - Seafood, some municipal drinking water

Iodine - Primarily iodized salt, seafoods, seaweeds

Manganese - Spinach, tea, rice, fruits

Copper - Lobster, oysters, avocados, fortified bran

Cobalt - Meats, dairy products, seafood

Selenium - Grains, bran, wheat germ, broccoli, clams

Chromium - Beer, beef, black pepper, some vegetables

Molybdenum - Cereals, buckwheat, tomato sauce

CHAPTER 7

Avoid Quacks and
Their Scare Tactics

I want to share my views on food and mineral supplements, "secret" nutrition formulas, and megavitamins with you for three reasons: (1) I am concerned that you might spend your money on something that is useless or even harmful; (2) some promoters might lead you to believe that no matter what you eat, you will still need their supplements; (3) others might try to convince you that you can eat anything you want, as long as you use their supplements.

Through saturation advertising, we have been led to believe that large doses of vitamins, minerals, and other products will do just about anything for us—anything from making our hair healthy to providing us with boundless energy. Look around you at the volume of newspaper, magazine, and TV ads which promote such products. The reason for such promotions is simple. This is approximately a $10-billion-a-year business.

A major fraud in the United States is the selling of pills, powders, potions, and supplements, instead of food, all in the name of good nutrition. Quacks who promote such items of "nutrition" do so for the revenue that it generates.

The pills, supplements, and diets which they promote range from the useless to the dangerous. Their scare tactics are simple. They falsely claim that people in the United States are dying faster than ever before because of the "bad" American diet—then they offer to sell their supplements to correct the "bad" diet. In fact, just the opposite is true; people are living longer than ever before. Life expectancy has increased significantly in the last decade. Life expectancy was approximately 50 years at the turn of the century. It is now well past 70, and is continuing to increase. It's interesting that these individuals who are so concerned about your "bad" diet don't tell you how you can correct your diet by eating the proper foods.

They know how to live off the anxiety of individuals. Another technique for selling is to ask a seemingly harmless question such as, "Is your diet, like that of so many others, vitamin deficient?" (Like so many others who live *where*?) The false premise that they are interjecting by asking such a question is that a great many people have vitamin-deficient diets. They don't—at least not in the United States.

Do we get enough A and C without taking vitamins?

The average American receives from his diet approximately 120 percent of the recommended daily allowance of vitamins A and C and is probably getting sufficient amounts of most of the other vitamins and minerals. Interestingly, the individuals to whom the scare tactics are directed are the very ones who would be the least likely to have vitamin or mineral deficiency. People who read about nutrition and buy supplements usually have an income and education level compatible with a lifestyle that would provide them with the very highest of nutrient intake. Still, it's been estimated that approximately half of all Americans take vitamin C supplements, and about half of the elderly take nutrition supplements of various types.

Those who disseminate misinformation have another type of false premise that they interject in order to promote their product. They will quote a *legitimate* scientific study which associates a reduced cancer risk with the ingestion of a certain vitamin or mineral, then they will offer that vitamin or mineral for sale as a supplement. What they don't tell the prospective buyer is that the scientific studies have always been done with *foods, not with supplements.* Responsible scientists know this. It is possible that the foods which were investigated and found to be responsible for the reduced cancer risk might have contained some substance other than the vitamin or mineral that was responsible for the reduced risk.

One final word about the use of the false premise. Some products will carry a "truthful" health claim and still convey the wrong message. By telling you that you need calcium—a truthful statement—and then telling you that their product contains calcium, they imply that you need more of their product. The same is true for products which contain other vitamins and minerals. The implication is that you need more of their product. Even though they make "truthful" claims, they do not convey the message that you should eat moderate amounts of a variety of foods. Neither does the truthful claim warn you of the dangers of excesses of certain vitamins and minerals.

People who would push supplements on you often use anecdotes and testimonials to "prove" that they *know* what is good for you. That reminds me of the humorist Josh Billings, who said, "The trouble with people isn't that they don't know, but that so much of what they know ain't so." Anecdotes and testimonials are not facts. Anecdotes and testimonials are not evidence—not even circumstantial evidence. They don't separate fact from fiction. They don't prove anything.

Even epidemiological studies, as valuable as they are, don't prove cause and effect. They can provide a lead for a new direction in research, can produce inferences, can provide circumstantial evidence, can give odds on there being a cause and effect, but they do not *prove* cause and effect. Scientific research and clinical trials prove cause and effect.

Do you recommend any vitamin or mineral supplements at all?

I recommend that you throw away all pills, supplements, potions, and megavitamins which have not been prescribed for you by your physician. Then you can concentrate on getting vitamins, minerals, trace elements, essential fatty acids, essential amino acids, and any other necessary nutrients from the foods that you eat.

I can just hear someone saying, "But where will I get my selenium, that substance that prevents cancer and slows the aging process?" I know of no studies which show that selenium protects a human against cancer or aging, but the body does need some selenium. If you are concerned about your selenium levels, eat some seafood—a bowl of clam chowder—or some bran, or broccoli.

Or someone might say, "But my large doses of vitamin E give me energy." Advertising claims aside, vitamins are not sources of energy. Besides, one scientific study showed that older individuals who took large doses of vitamin E died twice as fast as those who took no vitamin E (*Proceedings, National Academy of Sciences* 79:6023-6027, 1982). Promoters of food supplements and megavitamins often conveniently fail to mention such studies.

Keep the principle of moderation in mind when you consider what makes a healthy diet. Americans, for instance have been urged to reduce the calories that come from fat, not to eliminate fat completely. Here are some other examples which make a good case for the practice of moderation.

For example, suppose you feel you need some copper so that your bone marrow will be able to efficiently synthesize hemoglobin. You know that copper is found in avocados, oysters, lobsters, and fortified bran. That doesn't mean that you have to eat avocados, oysters, lobsters, and fortified bran every day. Occasionally eating one of them will provide enough copper. The same holds true for the other minerals.

Where does the need for fiber fit in?

Nutritionists urge us to eat fiber. Though no definitive studies have been done which *prove* that eating large quantities of fiber protects against colon cancer, it probably does. The recommendations are based on Burkitt's studies of natives in Africa who eat more fiber than Americans. They eat more fiber, but they have entirely different diets and do not get fiber from supermarket bran cereals. To prove that fiber is protective would require a long-term study of several thousand people who eat fiber and several thousand who do not, in order to determine the frequency of colon cancer in each group. A clinical trial of this type would show that fiber is beneficial or is not, or that it makes no difference. We can assume that it is beneficial for individuals to get between 15 and 35 grams of fiber a day, but more would not necessarily be better. Excessive dietary fiber may bind some essential minerals such as iron and zinc and prevent their absorption.

Is a vegetarian diet the answer to good health?

Many believe that a vegetarian diet is associated with increased longevity. We certainly should get the majority of our calories from complex carbohydrates, and vegetables do contain complex carbohydrates. But there has been no documentation that vegetarian diets result in increased longevity. That Seventh Day Adventists appear to live longer is often used as "evidence"—this is an example of anecdotal evidence—that a vegetarian diet will increase longevity. The Seventh Day Adventists and the Mormons apparently live longer than the average American because they do not smoke and they drink moderately, if at all. The Mormons consume more meat than the Seventh Day Adventists, and have a fairly high sugar consumption. Approximately half of the Seventh Day Adventists eat meat at intervals ranging from less than once a week to five or more times a week. Only two percent of them are vegan vegetarians. Claims that largely vegetarian diets will increase longevity should be examined in light of the "proof" that is offered to substantiate the claim. Until that time, think in terms of *variety* and *moderation* when it comes to diet.

Does a person on a reduced calorie diet need to take vitamins?

It is not necessary for people who are on diets with reduced caloric intakes to take vitamins or other supplements. If they eat foods from the different food groups and a variety of foods from within the various groups, they will have a balanced diet, even on an intake of 1,200 calories per day or less. One team of scientists (Duncan et al, *American Journal of Clinical Nutrition* 37:763-767, 1983) used a 1,000-calorie per day weight-loss diet for a period of six months. They selected a variety of foods, fed the foods in moderation, and made certain that the diet was a balanced one. They measured vitamin and mineral content in living tissue, and found that, during the period of the study, none of the vitamin or mineral levels fell.

Victor Herbert has written extensively about megavitamins, food fads, and quack nutrition (*Health Promotion and Disease Prevention in the Elderly*, Raven Press, Ltd., New York, 1988. See also references.) Herbert notes that, in addition to the megavitamins, food fads, and quack nutrition that are promoted, life extension potions, anti-aging elixirs and sex-rejuvenation frauds also abound. Here are two examples.

One "life extension" substance is Gerovital, the main ingredient of which is procaine. Procaine is a local anesthetic which may be useful to the physician or dentist, but it doesn't prevent aging. The breakdown product of procaine is para-aminobenzoic acid (PABA). Herbert notes that some American quacks have sold PABA as "anti-aging procaine tablets." PABA is a B-vitamin for bacteria (but not for humans). It is also a good sun blocker, but, as Herbert noted, it is unsafe to drink your suntan lotion.

Another "anti-aging" substance is ribonucleic acid (RNA). RNA not only isn't an anti-aging factor, it never gets into the bloodstream as

RNA. It is digested by intestinal enzymes, absorbed, and metabolized. There are many "anti-aging" substances. Among them are hormone supplements, herbal concoctions, dolomite, and lecithin. Another is fetal lamb tissue suspensions which are injected beneath the skin. These suspensions of cells are promptly destroyed and absorbed by the body, as are any other foreign cells.

Promoters of food supplements and megavitamins don't necessarily have our best interests at heart. Even if they believe that they do, it is *our* responsibility to take care of our health and assume the consequences of our actions. Then we can quit the age-old custom of oscillating between being "sick" and "well," and begin oscillating between being "well" and "exceptionally healthy."

We can increase our intake of vitamins and minerals, but not with commercial products. We can increase the intake of those substances by the judicious selection of food, and by lifestyle changes that will allow us to consume more calories.

Does this mean that vitamin or mineral supplements should never be taken?

No, it doesn't mean that at all. If you have anemia, a demonstrated vitamin or mineral deficiency, or some other medical problem, your physician might recommend that you increase your intake of a particular vitamin or mineral. If you are not eating a balanced diet, your physician will probably recommend that you begin doing so, or that you take a vitamin and/or mineral supplement. Otherwise, don't waste your time, money, and health on supplements.

There are millions of adults—estimates run as high as 40 million— who are taking megavitamin and mineral supplements in the belief that they will have more energy and improve their health. Despite the fact that a whole spectrum of individuals, from health professionals to athletic trainers, advocates the use of megavitamins, there is no scientific evidence that the people who take them are either healthier or more energetic than those who don't. Vitamins contain no usable energy. Scientifically minded health professionals know this. In fact, megavitamins can be harmful to one's health.

What happens to the excess vitamins that we consume?

Once a person consumes the vitamins that his body requires through the foods that he eats, the excess is either stored or excreted. The fat-soluble vitamins are stored, and the water-soluble vitamins are excreted, as are, for the most part, excess minerals. The process of excreting the extra vitamins and minerals that are obtained from *foods* isn't a problem for the kidneys. The process of excreting huge loads of vitamins and minerals as occurs when one takes megadoses of these substances, does put an additional work load on the kidneys. Also, the storage of excessive amounts of fat-soluble vitamins in the body is toxic.

The fat-soluble vitamins can be stored in the body for prolonged periods of time. For example, if you are healthy and well nourished, you have enough vitamin A stored in your liver to maintain you for a period of almost two years without any additional intake. Of course, no responsible person would recommend that you try going for two years without vitamin A. I am only pointing out the extent to which fat-soluble vitamins can be stored in the body. The quantity of vitamin D stored in the liver could probably maintain a person for up to five months. Not much is known about the storage of vitamin E, and the storage of vitamin K is slight. Still, megadoses of vitamins do not promote good health.

Are large doses of vitamins really all that bad for a person?

A number of subtle (or full-blown) medical symptoms can result from vitamin overdoses. For example, too much vitamin A can cause abdominal pain, fatigue, dermatitis, headaches, excessive irritability, hair loss, muscle pains, decalcification of bones, and edema (swelling).

An overdose of vitamin D can cause calcification of the soft tissue—blood vessels, heart, lungs—and leads to the formation of kidney stones. The daily requirement of vitamin D for a person eating a healthy diet can be met by exposure to the sun for five to ten minutes each day.

There are other adverse consequences of temporarily having high levels of the water-soluble vitamins in the body in addition to the burden on the kidneys. High doses of some of the B vitamins may cause nervous system dysfunctions, such as numbness of the feet and hands, as well as an impairment of other sensory functions.

Too much vitamin C interferes with the absorption of copper which can affect iron absorption and metabolism and produce iron deficiency anemia. A person could take large doses of vitamin C in the belief that it would energize him, only to have it do just the opposite. One of the first symptoms of anemia is fatigue.

There is another problem with this purely superstitious behavior of taking megadoses of vitamins and minerals: It deceives us. It shifts our attention in the wrong direction. It takes the emphasis off what is really important. What we really need for health, for preventing premature aging, and for energy is a sensible eating plan.

You will be doing yourself a real favor when you adopt a sensible eating and exercise plan. With such a plan you will increase your odds of living in good health to the very end of your life span. Further, you won't have to worry about whether or not megavitamins and mineral supplements are harming your body.

But is it not true that most of the people in the U.S. are deficient in one or more of the vitamins?

No, not really. Some are. Here's why.

The average person in the U.S. obtains about 40-50 percent of his calories from fats. Refined fats have few vitamins and minerals. Animal fats have some vitamins and minerals, but very few in comparison to the total number of calories that they contain. In addition, the average adult in the U.S. obtains about 600 of his calories from sugar each day. This explains why it is possible to have a vitamin deficiency on a caloric intake that is adequate. Compare the two diets below. Diet A is likely deficient in one or more of the vitamins. Diet B (assuming a variety of nutritious foods) contains more than an adequate supply of vitamins, minerals, and trace elements.

	Diet A	Diet B
Total calories	2,500	2,500
Fat calories	1,100 (44 percent)	375 (15 percent)
Sugar calories	600 (24 percent)	150 (6 percent)
Calories from vitamin and mineral foods	800	1,975

Though both diets supply 2,500 calories, that is where the similarity ends. The most striking difference lies in the number of calories supplied by foods which are rich in vitamins and minerals. The person on Diet A would get only 800 of his calories from such foods, while the person on diet B would get 1,975 of his calories from foods which are rich in vitamins and minerals. *The person on Diet B would be consuming more than twice as many vitamins and minerals as the person on Diet A,* and the source would be foods and not supplements. It isn't surprising that some people in the U.S. have an adequate, or more than adequate, intake of calories but still have a deficiency of one or more of the vitamins and/or minerals.

Two additional observations about Diet A and Diet B: (1) Adding megavitamins to Diet A doesn't make it as healthy as Diet B. (2) It isn't necessary to add megavitamins to Diet B.

People have asked me whether individuals who burn an extra 300 to 400 calories a day by exercising need more vitamins and minerals than those who do not exercise. My reply is that they are *already* getting additional vitamins and minerals when they increase their caloric intake, if they select the proper foods from which to get the extra calories. Remember, you may be able to more than double your intake of vitamins, minerals, and trace elements, without increasing your caloric intake, simply by eating vitamin-rich foods.

You don't need "secret" nutrition formulas, "new" food supplements, or expensive megavitamins in order to be healthy. As you begin to gravitate toward a diet similar to Diet B above, you will begin getting all of the vitamins and minerals that your body needs. Your body can then function at the very optimum level possible. You will have "long-term" vigor.

Should I feed my body this way permanently?

If you would like to increase your odds of enjoying good health to the very end of your life span, the answer is a resounding *yes*. Get into the habit of browsing through the produce section of your supermarket. Become accustomed to selecting a variety of fruits and vegetables to eat. Supplement these foods with complex carbohydrates (pastas, rice, etc.) and with grains and cereals. Feed your body this way permanently.

Why will I feel better if I feed my body this way permanently?

Human nature is such that mental and physical "feel-good-all-the-time" sensations come from *long-term* behaviors. For that reason, I believe you *will* feel good if you pursue the course of providing your body with the best nutrients possible on a permanent basis. (You will find that the foods which you select will taste better and better—to the extent that you will begin to perceive fat-laden foods as unpalatable.) As your long-term behavior changes, you will have more feel-good-all-the-time sensations. Let's explore this long-term-behavior concept a bit further, with regard to feeling good both mentally and physically.

Surges of good mental feelings can occur as a result of accomplishments such as winning an important match, receiving an honor, or winning a prize. This sort of experience raises the blood adrenalin levels and elevates the levels of endorphins in the body. The immediate event produces surges of good mental feelings, though it usually represents the culmination of a job well done over a long period of time.

How can I make these good feelings last?

As much as we would like for the surges of good feelings to last, they don't. When the adrenalin levels and the endorphin levels decrease, the feelings fade. Our feel-good-all-the-time sensations come from such accomplishments as doing our job well, making a contribution to our community, being a responsible person, contributing to the happiness and well-being of our family, believing that what we are doing has purpose, or having the will to make a small sacrifice now for a larger reward later. Both the surges of good mental feelings and the long-term good mental feelings are important. The same is true of our physical feelings. If we wake up some morning feeling unusually good, it might be because we did some aerobic exercise, had some healthy food, and got a good night's sleep. Almost everyone, even the chronically ill, feel better at some times than they do at others. We all have our "surges" of good physical feelings. But like our mental feelings, our physical day-in-and-day-out feel-good-all-the-time sensations come from constant attention to our health.

Can an old dog learn new tricks?

Without a doubt! Let us not think that we cannot change. Let us not think ourselves into being older than we are. Let us not think that our capabilities are less than they are. No one is going to do the changing for us. We are going to have to do it for ourselves. We are going to have to rewrite the script for our own lifestyle. The admonition "Physician, heal thyself" was never more appropriate than it is now. Just because a certain number of years have passed and we have reached a certain chronological age doesn't mean that we have to go into a state of artificial hibernation.

Summary

As we become healthier, we will feel better physically. As we feel better physically, we will feel happier. These things help prevent premature aging.

We can eliminate pills, supplements, megavitamins, potions, and similar substances which may do us harm. We can eliminate things like Gerovital and RNA pills. We can steer clear of procaine, herbal concoctions, and dolomite. *All of these things combined can't hold a candle to the effects of eating a variety of foods over a period of time, while paying careful attention to moderation and caloric balance.*

The seven United States Dietary Guidelines (USDA Bulletin HG232) are not flashy or exotic, but they will go much farther toward preventing premature aging than any of the fraudulent techniques discussed in this chapter. The seven U.S. Dietary Guidelines are:

1. *Eat a variety of foods.*
2. *Maintain a desirable weight.*
3. *Avoid too much fat, saturated fat, and cholesterol.*
4. *Eat foods with adequate starch and fiber.*
5. *Avoid too much sugar.*
6. *Avoid too much sodium.*
7. *If you drink alcoholic beverages, do so in moderation.*

CHAPTER 8

Enhancing "The Good Life" for Everyone

It will be enormously gratifying to me if the information in this book helps you to look younger, feel better, and live longer. Besides, if you live longer, that will probably help *me* to live longer. How can that be? As the life expectancy of large groups of people increases, the total storehouse of human knowledge and experience will automatically expand. That expansion of knowledge and experience will enhance "the good life" for everyone. Here's how:

The increase in human knowledge and experience will allow us to solve more problems. The ability to solve more problems will serve to further extend the human life expectancy and life span. The whole process will become self perpetuating. As we solve more problems, we will live longer, and as we live longer we will be able to solve more problems. Figure 1 on the following page shows an example of how the existing bulk of knowledge and experience can *now* be dramatically increased. In this example we consider 100,000 people in two different situations. In the first situation, the individuals grow and develop into adults, become educated and skilled in a trade or profession, and begin to use their talents at age 25. Soon thereafter their numbers begin to decrease as a result of deaths from diseases and accidents. The ones who survive use their skills until approximately the age of 65. Consequently, the area under the curve between the dotted lines represents the total contribution to the body of knowledge and experience of the original 100,000 people.

In the second situation, the people live longer. As deaths from diseases and accidents decrease, more people live to near the end of the human life span of 110 years. That changes the shape of the curve in Figure 1. The shaded area is added. The quantity of knowledge and experience which is gained is represented by that shaded area under the curve. If we take advantage of this vast new pool of knowledge and experience,

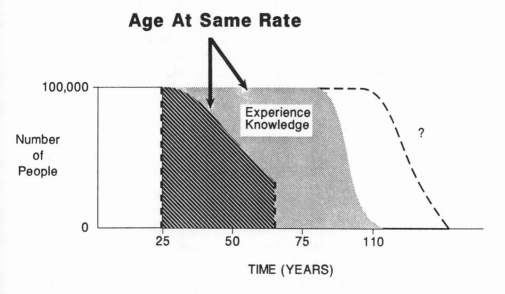

Figure 1. The extent to which the total body of human experience and knowledge can be expanded is shown.

we will have a significantly increased potential for problem solving. The shaded area under the curve is rapidly expanding. Each year it comes closer to the shape depicted in Figure 1.

We will soon have the problem-solving potential represented by the area between the dotted lines under the lower curve, *plus* the new problem-solving potential represented by the shaded area. The combination should produce some astonishing results. We are likely to see changes in every single facet of our lifestyle.

Let's examine something even more exciting. Suppose we are able to extend the human life span. If that happens, the curve will be extended as indicated by the dashed line in Figure 1. By the time we are able to do that, we surely will have learned to stop wasting one of our most valuable resources—the know-how of older people. We can begin expanding the body of knowledge and experience by understanding the meaning of "youth."

Is youth a state of being?

Yes, that's exactly what it is. Recently I talked to an individual who on her 65th birthday wanted to do something that she had never done before. Since she had always been alert, curious, and active, she had already tried many of the activities that are on her "things to do in this lifetime" list. One of the few things that she had never done was ride a motorcycle. She rode one on her 65th birthday, thought it was great fun, and will probably ride them again.

By coincidence, a few months after the motorcycle ride, she got married. Her family's analysis of the situation was that the exciting motorcycle ride made her feel young again, and made her decide to get married. The truth is, she has always been so involved with life that she has never *stopped* being young. That's probably the reason she looks approximately 15 years younger than her chronological age.

We have already seen how mental activity puts the aging process on hold. It is difficult to overstate the importance of that phenomenon. The person mentioned above has always been mentally active. She was a health professional during her "working" years. Even though she has retired from her first profession, she continues to be actively involved in developing home health care programs for her community. In addition to being mentally active, she is physically active. There is something to be learned here. A good balance of mental and physical activity is ideal. Let's examine the issue of physical activity from a perspective that is slightly different from the way that it is ordinarily analyzed.

Is there a prescription for inhibiting aging?

Yes, there is a miraculous prescription. It will make you look and feel younger; it will help you "unwind" at the end of the day; it will help cure your insomnia; it will increase your lean body mass and decrease your body fat stores; it will lower your resting heart rate; it will help lower your blood pressure; it will speed the flow of oxygen to all of the tissues of your body; it will let you consume some additional calories each day; it will decrease your need for tranquilizers; it will help you feel less fatigued during your regular daily activities; and it will help you to live longer. The prescription costs nothing and is available to everyone. I am talking about *aerobic exercise.*

So much has been written about the beneficial effects of aerobic exercise that it might seem as though nothing new could be said about it. Nevertheless, I would like for you to think about it this way: aerobic exercise will allow you to add additional, essential nutrients to your body and will help you to be healthier and live longer.

What exactly is aerobic exercise?

If you exercise at such a rate that you can breathe oxygen into your body as fast as you use it, you are doing an *aerobic* exercise. Walking, jogging, and playing tennis are all examples. If you exercise at such a rate that you use oxygen *faster* than you can breathe it into your body, you are doing an *anaerobic* exercise. A 100-yard dash is an example of an anaerobic exercise. If you run a 100-yard dash, at the end of the run you must breathe hard for a while in order to "pay back" the oxygen that you used while running.

Which aerobic exercise is the best?

The "best" is the one that is the best for you. Walking, bike riding, swimming, jogging, and organized exercise classes are all good aerobic activities. Obviously not all of them are available to everyone all the time.

Bike riding is fun, but one must have a bike and a safe place to ride. A stationary bike can be ridden year round, but it isn't easy to carry along on trips. Swimming requires a pool and may be seasonal. The amount of time an individual can spend jogging depends, among other things, on the weather and on the jogger's resistance to injury. Tennis, racquetball, rowing, and aerobics classes may depend on the availability of equipment and/or facilities. Engaging in a variety of aerobic exercises is probably the best approach.

For purposes of our discussion of aerobic exercise, we are going to use walking as the example. Walking is a universal activity requiring no special equipment; it doesn't promote injuries, isn't seasonal, and is a very effective aerobic exercise. (If you prefer a different aerobic exercise, that is okay. Just apply the same principles we will be applying to walking.)

Have walking and other aerobic exercises been proven effective?

For years scientists have suspected that aerobic exercise offers protection against coronary heart disease. We have seen how the Masai of Tanzania achieve an incredible degree of physical fitness—in some instances exceeding that of Olympic athletes—by walking every day. They do well despite a bad diet. Other studies have shown that conductors on London buses have a lower incidence of heart disease than do the drivers. Postmen who walk to deliver the mail have a lower incidence of heart disease than do the clerks who work in the offices. Studies of Dakota farmers and of Finnish lumberjacks suggest that physically active persons have less coronary heart disease than do inactive individuals.

It has now been established that *aerobic exercise increases life expectancy*. The type of exercise doesn't seem to matter—it can be anything from walking to participation in sports. Exercise apparently doesn't increase life expectancy *only* by decreasing the incidence of heart disease—although that would be reason enough to exercise. An excellent study has shown that exercise decreases death rates from *all causes* (Paffenbarger, 1986). The study, done on 16,000 men, showed that death rates decreased steadily as energy expended on aerobic exercises increased.

In Paffenbarger's study, death rates from all causes were one-fourth to one-third lower among those who expended an extra 2,000 calories a week. The older men at the highest level of activity had half the risk of those at the lowest level of activity. The men who were sedentary, even if they had once been varsity athletes, had a high risk of heart attack and stroke.

Keep the figure 2,000 in mind. In the discussion below we will focus on the importance of burning an extra 2,000 calories a week as a desirable goal.

How does exercise increase life expectancy?

The mechanisms by which exercise reduces the risk of death from *all* causes have not been worked out. Exercise lowers the blood pressure, decreases the heart rate, lowers the level of the harmful low-density lipoproteins in the blood, and raises the level of the beneficial high-density lipoproteins in the blood. By lowering the blood-lipid (fat) level, exercise decreases the rate of development of hardening of the arteries. Exercise gives the respiratory system a workout and speeds the flow of oxygen to all of the tissues of the body. Exercise increases the lean body mass and decreases the fat stores of the body. Exercise keeps the entire organism more alert and less fatigued. All of these factors contribute to the exercise-induced increase in life expectancy, but there are other factors which should receive attention: Exercise makes a person feel good about himself. It makes a person feel better today than he did yesterday and it helps him to feel that he has conquered laziness. In short, exercise sends a flood of good self-esteem signals to the subconscious mind. Also, individuals who exercise tend to eat healthier foods than do sedentary people, and because they exercise, they eat *larger quantities* of those healthy foods.

You are now in a position to take advantage of two known facts:

1. *Physical fitness increases life expectancy.*
2. *Walking is an excellent way to become physically fit.*

Is walking really that good for me?

You can enhance your lifestyle, decrease your level of fatigue, increase your intake of healthy foods, look and feel younger, and increase your life expectancy by walking an extra three miles each day. It isn't necessary for you to walk three miles a day in order to achieve cardiovascular fitness. You can do that by walking (briskly) 30 minutes a day, four days a week. I would encourage you to walk three miles a day so you can get above the 2,000-calories-a-week level—the level that Paffenbarger found would decrease death rates from *all* causes. Also, when you walk three miles a day, you can add an extra 2,000 calories of nutrient-dense foods to your weekly diet. That will give your body a wonderful array of vitamins, minerals, and trace elements with which to maintain, replace, and repair the cells in your body. Yes, walking really *is* that good for you!

How fast should I walk?

Your walk should be moderately paced and relaxed. If you have been sedentary for a while, you will probably need to begin by walking slowly for short distances. Then you can gradually work up to a faster pace and longer distances. You might start out by walking a mile over a period of 25 to 30 minutes. As you become stronger, you will be able to walk faster, for longer distances. You might eventually work up to a 15-minutes-per-mile pace. Many people do. Some get up to a 12-minutes-per-mile pace—a pace equivalent to a slow jog. It isn't necessary to strive for that speed in order to derive the benefits from walking. Just walk at a good pace, swing your arms freely, and don't slump over as you walk. Don't try to make your strides too long. A good pair of walking or running shoes will make your walk more comfortable. Your walk should be continuous so that you'll keep your heart rate elevated for a significant period of time.

Once you work up to a 15-minutes-per-mile pace, you will be able to get in your daily walks in 45 minutes. Don't push yourself too hard. If while walking you are exerting yourself so much that you are unable to carry on a conversation with someone, slow down just a bit. Walk at a good, brisk pace just below that level of exertion. That will be a fast enough rate to elevate your heart rate to a desirable level.

How can I know my heart rate has reached a desirable level?

If you want to be more precise in maintaining an ideal heart rate while you walk, subtract your age from 220. Then during your walk, get your heart rate up to 70 percent of that number. For example if you are 50 years old, the calculations would be as follows: $220 - 50 = 170$, and 70 percent of $170 = 119$. In this instance you would want your heart rate to get up to approximately 120 beats per minute (but not over 136 beats per minute, which is 80 percent of 170).

It is okay to calculate what your pulse rate should be while you walk, but it is probably simpler just to walk at a good hard pace. Obviously, as you become more physically fit, your walking will become easier, and you will need to pick up your pace in order to get your heart rate up. (Note: If you prefer to burn your 2,000 calories per week doing some other type of aerobic activity, the same principles regarding pulse rate apply. Perform at a sufficient level to elevate your pulse rate to the range indicated by the calculations above.)

What if I just don't have time to exercise?

It's easy to think that you don't have time—even 45 minutes a day—to fit aerobic exercise into your daily schedule. Remind yourself, though, that seeing to your health and working toward increasing your longevity are as important as anything else that you could do with your time. Once your family and friends understand that, they are likely to be supportive of your efforts.

There is no reason to think that you are indulging yourself (or wasting time) by exercising, when you could be doing something "more constructive." *Exercise won't take time from you, it will give time to you by giving you the energy to accomplish more in less time.* If you are a very busy person, you are the one who needs the exercise the most. If exercise will give you more of that precious commodity called time, that alone is reason enough for exercising. Most of us probably fritter away enough time each day to do all of the exercising necessary to keep us healthy.

Who has the most time for exercising? Let me quote Arnold Bennett (*How to Live on 24 Hours a Day,* by permission of Doubleday, Doran & Co., 1910):

> Philosophers have explained space. They have not explained time. It is the inexplicable raw material of everything. With it, all is possible; without it, nothing. The supply of time is truly a daily miracle....You wake up in the morning, and lo! your purse is magically filled with 24 hours of the unmanufactured tissue of the universe of your life! It is yours....No one can take it from you. It is unstealable. And no one receives either more or less than you receive....In the realm of time there is no aristocracy of wealth, and no aristocracy of intellect. Genius is never rewarded by even an extra hour a day. And there is no punishment. Waste your infinitely precious commodity as much as you will, and the supply will never be withheld from you....Moreover, you cannot draw on the future. Impossible to get into debt! You can only waste the passing moment. You cannot waste tomorrow; it is kept for you. You cannot waste the next hour; it is kept for you....You have to live on this 24 hours of daily time....Money is far more common than time. When one reflects, one perceives that money is just about the most common thing there is....The supply of time, though gloriously regular, is cruelly restricted....Which of us is not saying to himself—which of us has not been saying to himself all his life: ''I shall alter that when

I have a little more time''? We never shall have any more time. We have, and we have always had, all the time there is.

Maybe it is reassuring to know that more time is not allotted to the wealthy, or to the genius, or to the holder of the highest title. On the other hand, it *is* possible to obtain more time for ourselves. Paffenbarger's study has shown that exercise gives individuals more time because it decreases the death rate from all causes. Also, exercise gives individuals more time by making them energetic enough to do more in less time. Perhaps the person who can't wait to get out there and engage in some type of aerobic exercise is subconsciously aware of this. Anything that a person could do to more completely fill, or enrich, the time available to him would certainly seem to be worth doing.

Let us not lose sight of our goal—to maintain a state of super health and youthfulness right to the end of our life span—and then perhaps see the life span extended. When we burn an extra 2,000 calories a week, that means that each week we can eat an extra 2,000 calories of vitamin-rich foods *in addition to our regular caloric intake*. That will allow the vitamins and minerals contained in those foods to permeate the fluids which bathe the cells of our bodies, thus keeping the cells healthy, and helping us toward the goals mentioned above.

We want to get all of the time that is coming to us—all 110 years, and then some. We want to enjoy that time in the best possible fashion. But we must keep our mind on our goal. We don't want to find, as Santayana said, that we have "redoubled our efforts now that we have lost sight of our goal."

Will becoming creative inhibit aging?

Yes, many geniuses have shown that the creative process is one of the most significant age-inhibitors in existence, but you don't have to be a genius to be creative. Walking or other aerobic exercise will release the brakes on the creative process in both the conscious and the subconscious mind.

How do you know when the creative process is at work? As you get into walking, you will eventually cover a mile or two miles of a route that you walk every day and suddenly discover that you don't remember having passed certain familiar landmarks along the way. That is an indication that you have fully released the brakes on your thought processes, that you have begun to search in a creative fashion for new ideas or for solutions to problems. You are then in a truly creative "state." In such a state, your subconscious goal-seeking mechanisms can work on ways to move you toward other goals which you wish to achieve.

Students who fret with a mathematical problem or other problems commonly experience this phenomenon. When they take a break, play a game, go for a walk, or even go to sleep, the solution to the problem often comes to them. The common denominator in all of this is that the subconscious goal-seeking mechanism has a mission (the solution to the problem), and the goal-seeking mechanism will run impulses across as many neural circuits as necessary in order to achieve that goal.

If you have given your subconscious mind the charge to make you look, think, act, and feel as youthful, healthy, and energetic as possible, the millions of neural circuits in your brain will search for ways to achieve that goal. There is no better time for those circuits to become active than when you are completely immersed in an aerobic exercise.

Physical exercise and mental exercise, both of which are essential to inhibiting the aging processss, occur simultaneously when a person is really "into" an aerobic activity. The triple effect of burning calories, becoming more energetic, and becoming more creative serves to infuse an aliveness into a person. That person characteristically continues to exercise on a regular basis once he feels the addictive effect of the aliveness.

Can exercise influence feelings and emotions?

That is another beneficial aspect of physical exercise. The individual learns that he can't always control situations that cause him to *have* certain feelings—depression, for example—but he learns that he *can* control his *actions*. Controlling his actions exerts an influence on the way he feels. He uses this to his advantage. He engages in an aerobic activity, takes the brakes off his creative processes, and allows his creative processes to help him change the way he feels.

Will more exercise do more good?

It will certainly do more good for the creative process. I know individuals who frequently go for extra long walks, runs, or bike rides.

They want to "get the blood pumping," or "burn some extra calories," or "really clean out the system." I call these episodes of prolonged exercise "megaburns" because a lot of calories are used—more than is necessary for physical fitness. Doing megaburns allows one to eat more food, but that is probably not the reason for doing them. I think people do them because prolonged periods of aerobic exercise really do take the brakes off the creative process. Such a period gives the brain an opportunity to work without restraint. If two people talk while they walk, that conversation is likely to be much more creative than if the same two people sit in comfortable chairs facing each other. As you get into the habit of walking, you may be tempted sometimes to do megaburns. On some particular day, it will seem natural to walk farther than you would ordinarily walk. If you feel the urge, do it.

What does aerobic exercise do to our thought processes?

Whether or not you occasionally do megaburns, once you really become involved with an aerobic activity, you will eventually notice a change in your thought processes. Once your habit of daily walking is well established, you will find it easier to fall into a creative "trance." While in the trance, you will continue to be aware of pedestrians, automobiles, and obstacles to be avoided, yet creative thoughts will be running freely through your subconscious mind.

Since you have a goal-seeking mechanism built into your subconscious mind, one of these trance-like states is a good time to feed in new goals. Tell your goal-seeking mechanism that you feel stronger, healthier, happier, younger, more poised, more confident, or that you no longer smoke cigarettes, or any other thing else that you wish to feel, be, or do. *Feed in one goal at a time.* If those messages are fed into your goal-seeking mechanism enough times, the billions of neurons in your brain will busily seek ways to achieve those goals for you. If you will give this your best effort for at least one month, you will find that the only mistake I have made in presenting this information to you is that I understated the effectiveness of it.

Now, let's get down to some practicalities. When you activate your creative processes, you activate a significant inhibitor of the aging process. Aerobic exercises such as walking help you to get into a position to activate your creative processes. Also, your normal daily activities, *plus* the walking or other exercises that you do, will make it necessary for you to eat more food than you would ordinarily eat. *If you plan to enjoy optimum good health, it is essential that all of your calories come from quality food sources.*

Does quality food have to come from health food stores?

Absolutely not. The fresh produce section of your supermarket is an excellent place to find quality food, as are the canned and frozen fruit and vegetable sections.

One of the first things an exercising person does is examine his diet. Many get on a "health-food-store kick," and it isn't necessary. (For a more detailed discussion of this subject, see Susan R. Holman's, *Essentials of Nutrition*, pp. 162-167, Lippincott, Philadelphia, 1987.)

Advertising claims aside, foods from a health food store are not more nutritious than foods from a supermarket, and identical foods are almost always much more expensive in the health food store. It is certainly a person's prerogative to purchase his food anywhere he wishes, but he should know that the supermarket foods are just as nutritious as foods found in specialty stores. They are also usually just as chemical-free. This should be good news to the frugal individual or to the person with limited financial resources.

Salespersons in health food stores often claim that most people don't eat properly, and then recommend a supplement to balance the diet and prevent deficiencies. Unfortunately, they don't seem interested in teaching individuals how to select nutritionally adequate foods. It's ironic that the health food store is *not* always a good place to learn about good nutrition.

According to Holman, "Books and magazines may be sold that teach and promote current health fads. Authors often have degrees and training that sound credible, but that may not stand up under careful inspection. Many authors are 'directors' or 'doctors' of their own 'nutrition institutes.'"

Many health food stores do sell large quantities of food. You might find these stores helpful if you are looking for an unusual or foreign food, or for odd spices. But a good dose of skepticism can go a long way toward repelling some of the unfounded claims to which you might be subjected there.

What about additives?

You might be told that additives are "bad," when in fact, some preservatives such as acetic acid, sugar, citric acid, and antioxidants are naturally occurring substances. Preservatives make it possible to transport foods without spoilage and thus allow people to have balanced diets in all climates year round. Foods in health food stores may be advertised as being free of chemicals, even though studies have shown that residues in soil or wind may result in the same levels of chemicals in these foods as in the supermarket foods.

Are "natural" vitamins better than other kinds?

Claims are sometimes made that "natural" vitamins which are sold in the stores are better than synthesized vitamins, but since the vitamins from both sources have identical chemical structures, the body cannot tell the difference. The truth of the matter is that, although the individual making the claims might be sincere, there is no objective, scientifically tested evidence to support claims such as these. Legitimate claims can be supported with reports from the Food and Drug Administration, the National Cancer Institute, the United States Department of Agriculture, or a reprint of a published research article from a *legitimate* medical journal. If the advertising claims sound too good, ask for some legitimate supporting evidence. Here are some guidelines:

1. Long-term studies have *not* shown that "organic" foods from a health food store are either safer or more nutritious than foods grown with commercial fertilizers.

2. People who buy from the health food store more often than they buy from the supermarket are spending more money than is necessary for good nutrition (Holman, p.167).

3. An individual's food dollar will buy more of a variety of nutritious foods at the supermarket than that same dollar will buy at a health food store.

4. You are more likely to consume a rich supply of vitamins, minerals, and trace elements when you consume a large variety of foods.

Will longevity enhance the good life?

Longevity, which is coupled with continued health and vigor, is dependent upon the efficiency of the metabolic machinery in the body.

Increasing the efficiency of the metabolic machinery will enhance the good life.

This subject is dealt with more extensively in later sections of this book. It is raised here to make the point that when we are able to further manipulate diets to our advantage, the diets will still have to contain adequate quantities of the essential nutrients. The essential nutrients will always go a long way toward enhancing the good life.

Do our lifestyles affect our health?

Let's take a panoramic view. If we are going to make an effort to be super healthy—as opposed to just being "not sick"—we need to have an overall view of good health. It is sometimes easy to forget this and key in on one area (such as heart and blood vessel disease) while neglecting the others. The lifestyles of individuals are responsible for about one-half of the deaths in the United States. People are becoming more aware of that fact.

Corporations are also beginning to take note of this fact. Many are expanding their fitness programs into total health programs. In addition to encouraging fitness among their employees, many corporations have programs to aid in the detection and control of high blood pressure, to help eliminate alcohol and drug abuse as well as tobacco use, and to help reduce stress. Programs have been established for weight control and for early cancer detection. The corporations find that they can set up low-cost programs in conjunction with local nonprofit organizations such as the American Heart Association, the American Lung Association, or other agencies which are committed to total health care.

The panoramic approach to superior health and increased longevity is graphically shown in Figure 2. Superior health and increased longevity are shown at the hub of a wheel. The wheel has several spokes. Increasing human longevity can be enhanced *by attention to each spoke on the wheel*. Heart and blood vessel disease is shown on one spoke, weight control on another, and nutrition on another. Other spokes include: aerobic exercise, elimination of physical and mental stress, quitting smoking, eliminating alcohol and drug abuse, cancer detection, and accident prevention.

Obviously, several of the factors listed interact with each other. For example, good nutrition will go a long way toward preventing heart

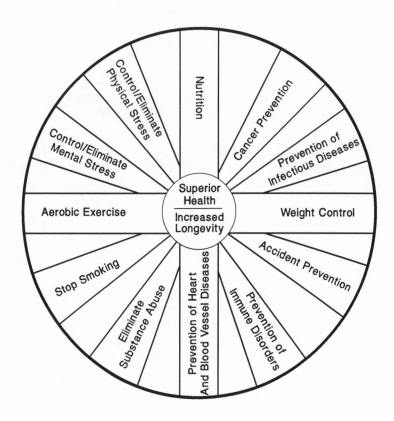

Figure 2. This figure shows that superior health and increased longevity involve a number of factors.

and blood vessel disease. Weight control and aerobic exercise will help to eliminate mental and physical stress and will help to prevent heart and blood vessel disease. Quitting smoking will allow one to do more aerobic exercise, the increased exercise will help control weight, the weight control and the exercise will help the heart, and so on. As you can see, there are numerous possibilities for interaction. Attention to all of the factors depicted by the spokes of the wheel will provide a synergistic effect on life expectancy. It makes the "whole" more than the sum of its parts.

If health has been neglected, how do we get on the road back to health?

Suppose an individual has completely neglected his mental and physical health so that all of the spokes on his health and longevity wheel need attention. The prospect of dealing with all of them at once may seem overwhelming. Yet the very fact that one spoke influences the others makes it possible to begin on only one of the spokes.

A physician may say to a patient, "Quit smoking, get some exercise, and lose 40 pounds." That might be good advice, but it seldom works. It would be more effective for the physician to say, "Spend a few minutes on an exercise bike each day. Gradually increase the length of your workouts until you attain a good level of physical fitness."

As the patient begins to concentrate on becoming physically fit, he is more likely to give up smoking and to lose weight. As he loses weight, he will probably develop an interest in good nutrition, and that interest will lead to....Well, you get the picture. He will ultimately be paying meticulous attention to his *total* health.

As our hypothetical patient begins to pay attention to more and more spokes on the wheel, a synergistic effect on his health and life expectancy will be evident. He will feel better physically since his health is improving. He will feel better mentally and be happier because he is working toward a worthy goal. The simple act of beginning to spend a few minutes each day exercising will start him on the road to improvement. Spending a few minutes each day exercising will help him to know that he *can* achieve excellent health.

How important is mental attitude?

It is a known fact that one's health can be strengthened or weakened by his mental attitude. A person's attitude might make the difference between maintaining good health or losing it completely. If he begins the road to improvement by concentrating on changing only one facet of his lifestyle at a time, he will be more likely to continue down that road, and and less likely to make excuses for not continuing down it. He will feel good if he isn't put into a position of having to offer excuses to himself, or to someone else, for not working toward his goal. Making excuses might ease the pain of not completing the job, but it won't get the job done.

Suppose you want your joints to become more flexible, your muscles stronger, and your skin healthier and younger. Suppose you want your heart and lungs to be in better condition, you want to lose some weight, you want to quit smoking, you want to eliminate stress, you want to begin eating more nutritious food, and you want to begin a program of aerobic exercise. In other words, suppose you want to turn back the clock so that you can look and feel 10 years younger. What is the best way to begin? I am convinced that the best way to begin is to select one facet of your current lifestyle that you wish to change—*one that you are reasonably sure of succeeding at changing*, and put all your effort into changing *that one*.

Summary

Having chosen one aspect of your lifestyle to change, be a little arrogant about your chances of success. As you work on making the change, repeatedly say to yourself, "I am going to celebrate the change. I am going to celebrate the new me. I am not going to criticize myself or make excuses for my failures." One success will lead to another and then another, and then another. You will find that it isn't so much what needs to be changed that matters but the way that you *think* about what needs to be changed.

One success will infuse you with the enthusiasm and energy to make other changes in your lifestyle. As your enthusiasm grows, your blood level of endorphins will increase, your circulation will improve, and you will have more energy, vitality, and endurance. You will have more of that "energy of life" that was discussed earlier. You will indeed begin to look and feel younger.

CHAPTER 9

What Are Our Ultimate Biological Limits?

I recently saw a documentary film about the people in the Andean villages of Ecuador (see references). Some of the people who were interviewed on camera claimed to be 120 to 130 years old and older. These claims, though confirmed by church records, are questionable, but it is a fact that these people live to be very old. We just might learn something from these "primitive" people about extending our own life expectancy. Scientists who have studied them report that the percentage of centenarians in that population is many times that found in the United States.

Several influences affect the life expectancy of the Andean villagers. Old people in that area continue to be an important part of the society. They are expected to continue to work and carry their share of the load for as long as they live; they don't have a time in life to "retire." Further, the younger members of the society look up to them and expect them to be wise.

It is said that they don't seem to mind reaching an old age because, once they do, they have really "arrived." They are then members of that unique group of people who are respected and admired for their position in society and for their wisdom. Several generations of family members look up to them.

Maybe the aging clock of the Andeans does move at a slower rate than it does in people in some other societies. That isn't inconceivable. The aging clock of some people *within* the various societies of the world moves at a slower rate than it does in other people in those societies. If the Andeans have any "bad" genes to cause premature aging, the bad genes don't seem to work.

The diet of the Andeans who live in the mountain regions might seem sparse by some standards. They don't eat very much meat. Scientists who have studied them have found that their diet consists of approximately 15 percent protein, 15 percent fat, and 70 percent carbohydrate.

If these mountain dwellers want to go somewhere, they walk, either to the village or to visit someone, and this can mean walking half a day. They walk everywhere. They walk every day. They also—young, old, even those who are supposedly more than 100 years of age—engage in hard physical labor every day. We have seen how beneficial this sort of daily exercise is.

Can moderate fitness offer major protection?

With each passing day, additional evidence accumulates that exercise, even of a moderate nature, reduces death rates from heart disease. At an American Heart Association conference in Sante Fe, New Mexico (March, 1988), Dr. Harold Kohl presented the results of an eight-year study of 17,337 patients by the Institute for Aerobic Research in Dallas. The patients' average age was 45, they had normal ECG's, and none had evidence of heart disease.

Despite other risk factors such as blood pressure, cholesterol, and age, the effect of exercise was significant. The least fit men—those in the bottom 20 percent for physical fitness—had a death rate three times higher than men who were *moderately* fit (who fell in the 21 to 40 percentile range in fitness ratings). Women in the bottom 20 percent for fitness had a 73 percent higher death rate than those who were in the (moderate) 21 to 40 percentile range in fitness ratings. Dr. Kohl says, "In other words, just a bit more activity goes a long way—you don't need to run a marathon."

Maybe you don't need to run a marathon, but, as the saying goes, "If you're gonna dance, you've gotta pay the fiddler." If you're going to derive any benefit from exercise, you have to do it yourself. There are three things about exercise which appeal to me. First, no matter how wealthy you are, you can't derive any benefit whatsoever from exercise by hiring someone to do it for you. Second, whether you're rich, poor, or in between, you can't derive any benefit from exercise or exercise gadgets unless you have the self-discipline and motivation to get out there and do it yourself. Exercise doesn't have to be a chore. It can and should be fun, *but you still have to do it.* The third thing that makes exercise appealing is the feeling it gives that it is possible to cope with laziness and procrastination.

Do people in non-industrialized countries live longer than people in the U.S.?

Factors other than fitness and diet influence the longevity of people in different countries. One such factor may be emotional stress. It seems to be the consensus in some scientific circles that individuals in industrialized countries are subjected to more emotional stress than are people in nonindustrialized countries. I have serious doubts about that. That isn't an easy judgment to make. A stimulus that is a stressor for one person is not necessarily a stressor for another. A corporate executive might be even *more* stressed if he had to leave his office, walk around the mountains of Ecuador, eat fruit and vegetables, and do hard physical labor.

In the United States, too, most older people remain active. Many are also economically self-sufficient. More and more older individuals are continuing to make a contribution to society long after they "retire." Unfortunately, our image of an older person is often the image of a person who is needy and/or in poor health. That is a distorted view. It just doesn't fit the majority of the people in that age group in the United States. In fact, older people who remain vigorous, healthy, and self-sufficient are doing much to make ours an age-irrelevant society.

If you are talking to someone on the phone whom you have never met, and he tells you that he is 65 years old, that doesn't tell you anything at all about him except that he has lived for 65 years. He might be in excellent physical condition. Maybe his children are educated, and he has time (and more money) for other things. (The travel industry, in particular, has been influenced by older people.) Perhaps he is enrolled in formal education courses and is in the process of changing careers. He might not be in need of special health or social services—only 15 percent of those over 65 do need them. His aging clock might be moving at a very slow rate. He might be one of those individuals who is going to test the ultimate human biological limits.

In 1988, I spoke by phone to Mr. William McDaniel of Bay Springs, Mississippi. He told me that he felt fine, except that he couldn't see or hear as well as he once could, and that he has some problems with arthritis which started "a couple of years ago." All in all he sounded quite well for an individual who is in the process of testing his biological limits—he celebrated his 110th birthday on May 20, 1988.

Aging clocks move at different rates, and apparently McDaniel's has moved slowly for the past century. He thinks that his longevity is due, in part, to hard work, which included working on the railroad, and as a carpenter, blacksmith, auto mechanic, and brick mason. "Probably built more chimneys than any man that ever lived," he said. He also climbed a nearby fire tower at the age of 101. I asked him if he felt old. "A little," he replied.

Does hard work contribute to longevity?

Hard work very likely did contribute to McDaniel's longevity. People who live a long time usually do work hard. They also eat a balanced diet, get adequate sleep, maintain normal body weight, don't smoke, and drink in moderation—if at all. In fact, individuals who practice all of these health habits can expect to live ten to twelve years longer than those who don't practice them.

Health and longevity are more than just a continuing battle between disease processes and the body's defense mechanisms. Thought processes, attitudes, emotions, and the process of coping with an ever-changing world all interact to enhance or inhibit our health and longevity.

Do illnesses come from our minds?

The mechanisms by which thought processes might affect health and longevity have not been adequately studied. There are several reasons for this, not the least of which is the attitude of some health professionals. Recently, while I was having lunch with a group of physicians, one of them, a psychiatrist, made a statement which provoked a spirited debate. He said, "All of the diseases which exist originate in the minds of people. People have diseases because they 'think' themselves into having them." Maybe he believed the statement, or maybe he just wanted to provoke a discussion. I don't know. I do know that if the statement is true, the Salk vaccine certainly changed our mental attitude about polio.

Some people do believe that *all* diseases are "all in the mind." Many of those same individuals also believe that if a person with a disease assumes the proper mental attitude, the disease will go away. Unfortunately, this kind of thinking is one reason the effects of brain function and mental processes on health have not been adequately studied, nor well accepted.

How does the brain influence aging?

The brain certainly is important in maintaining health and longevity. Everything from preparing a grocery list to maintaining hormone production is managed by the brain. Because of the brain, stress can affect the heart and other organs of the body. The various organs of the body cannot perceive stress; but the brain can perceive it and send out signals which affect the entire body. This is possible because nerves innervate essentially every part of the body, and because neurotransmitters can transmit messages to all parts of the body.

A neurotransmitter is a substance that transmits nerve impulses from one nerve to another (across a synapse), or that transmits an impulse from a nerve to a target organ. Because the brain produces hundreds of neurotransmitters, it can affect the function of all of the organs of the body. Acetylcholine, norepinephrine, dopamine, and serotonin are all natural neurotransmitters. Beta endorphin and all of the other endorphins are also neurotransmitters. All of these substances make it possible for the brain to communicate with the body and to influence every function of the body. The brain can influence the cardiovascular, digestive, endocrine, muscular, respiratory, urinary, reproductive, integumentary (skin), and immune systems. The brain can influence secretion, excretion, and metabolism. Emotions, pain, mood, and thought are all products of brain function.

Will we be younger if we think younger?

The brain tends to perform according to the signals that it receives. People who live to the end of their life span likely don't look into the mirror every morning and say (or think), "I'm getting older." William McDaniel, because he was preoccupied with hard physical labor, likely didn't look into the mirror every morning and say, "I'm getting older." (One has to wonder what would happen to people like McDaniel if they looked into the mirror every morning and said, "I'm getting younger.")

A person's brain continually works to protect him. It works to maintain health or to restore it. Because the 100 billion or so cells of the brain are continually seeking ways to do this, suggesting beliefs to a receptive brain can cause shifts in mental and physiological function. If a person isn't going to suggest to his brain that he is young and healthy, at least he shouldn't suggest to it that he is old and sick.

If you tell an individual that he looks sick often enough, he will very likely begin to look, feel, act, and *be* sick. The same thing happens if you repeatedly tell a person that he is old, or if he repeatedly tells himself that he is old. He will begin to look, feel, act, and *be* old. That's one reason people in times past got old at the age of 50. They thought they were *supposed* to be old at that age.

How does the immune system influence aging?

Some who study the aging process believe that the immune system influences the rate at which a person ages. The immune system manufactures antibodies to protect the body from foreign invaders, but it does more. As the surface of the cells of the body changes, the immune system turns against the cells of its own body. The more the surface of the cell changes, the more rapidly the immune system forms antibodies to attack the body's own cells. An impaired immune system might attack the body's own cells prematurely.

Does the brain affect the immune system?

The brain can modulate the activity of the immune system. Extensive networks of nerves have been found in the lymph nodes, thymus gland, spleen, and bone marrow—the structures which comprise the immune system. The nerve networks and the neurotransmitters are the means by which the brain influences the activity of the immune system. Even if nerve networks and neurotransmitters had not been discovered, we would have known that the brain function affects the immune system. Long ago, Selye showed that stress causes the thymus gland, spleen, and lymph nodes to atrophy (Selye, H., *The Stress of Life,* New York, McGraw-Hill Book Co.).

We would have known that the brain influences the immune system because emotions such as depression and grief will lower the activity of T-lymphocytes, a type of white blood cell that attacks foreign invaders. Further, people who are subjected to undue stress have more fevers, an indication that they are more susceptible to infection; they also have more rashes, and their wounds heal at a slower rate. These pathological changes indicate that the overall immunity is decreased. Since the brain affects the way the immune system operates, it can change the susceptibility to certain diseases and can influence the rate at which one ages.

Is it possible to predict a person's future health?

If you were faced with trying to predict the future health of a large group of individuals, how would you go about doing it? Would it seem reasonable to first get a medical history and do a physical examination? That could be followed by X-rays and a series of clinical and laboratory tests. The results of the tests could be used to group the people according to whether they had excellent, good, fair, or poor health. That would be one way of predicting the future health of a large group of people.

Actually, there is a better way. You could simply ask them to rate their overall health. That would certainly be less expensive. More importantly, the results of a well-designed scientific study indicate that asking patients to rate their overall health might be *more accurate* than clinical examinations in predicting the future health of large groups of people.

Mossey and Shapiro (*American Journal of Public Health* 72:800, 1982) conducted such a study. Their investigation involved 3,500 elderly people and extended over a period of seven years. Objective health of the subjects was assessed by physicians. The subjects were also asked the following question: ''For your age, would you say in general your health is excellent, good, fair, poor, or bad?'' Those who rated their health as poor were almost three times more likely to die during the seven-year period of the study than those who rated their health as excellent. The subjects' perception of their health was more accurate in predicting who would die than were the objective health assessments as determined by the physicians. It probably isn't unusual for a person who is in poor health to know that he is in poor health. A more interesting finding which the study revealed is the fact that those individuals who *were* in poor health according to the physicians' tests survived at a higher rate, *as long as they believed their own health to be good.*

I am fully aware that our overall health is affected by a number of factors, such as infectious diseases, degenerative diseases, genes, access to health care, socioeconomic status, diet, emotional well-being, and body weight. Being aware of such factors should not prevent our utilizing the enormous power of the brain to help maintain our health and increase our longevity. I am firmly convinced that one reason some people live so long, and live in good health, is that they *expect* to do so.

Is there evidence that we can think ourselves well?

We have long suspected that perceptions and expectations influence one's health. That has now been scientifically documented in part by studying the effects of placebos.

A placebo is an inactive compound that may be given to a patient to satisfy that patient's perceived need for drug therapy. Placebos are also useful when there is a new drug to be tested or when an existing drug is to be tested on a new disease. Here's how that works:

If you developed a pill that you believed would be an effective treatment for hay fever, you could test it by giving it to 100 people with hay fever. To further demonstrate the effectiveness of the new pill, you could give a sugar pill, a placebo, to an additional 100 people with hay fever. Suppose your new pill worked. Suppose most of the people with hay fever were cured. Would it surprise you if some of the people who took the sugar pill—some who *thought* they were getting the new pill—were also cured? Well, that often happens, and it doesn't mean that the new pill was ineffective. The phenomenon is known as the "placebo effect."

Do those individuals who take the placebos just *think* they get better, or is there actual improvement? In many cases, according to laboratory and clinical tests, there is actual improvement. In controlled studies, placebos have been shown to have a beneficial effect on pain, nausea, asthma, acne, headaches, seasickness, and countless other disorders.

The brain, as we have seen, modulates the activity of the immune system and all of the other systems of the body. Also, the brain, with its network of nerves and neurotransmitters, communicates with virtually every cell in the body. In addition, the "thinking" part of the brain can send signals to the hypothalamus, an area on the underside of the brain. The hypothalamus can, in turn, signal the pituitary gland—the so-called master gland of the body—to release a multitude of hormones. These hormones control the powerful endocrine system, which is another master regulator of all of the body functions.

What can emotions do to our bodies?

Emotions such as ecstasy and expectation may (1) enhance the function of the immune system; (2) change the rate of production of the neurotransmitters; and (3) stimulate the hypothalamus to signal the pituitary gland to release hormones.

These are the mechanisms by which placebos produce measurable improvements in some conditions. On the other hand, placebos can adversely affect the body. If you gave a sugar pill to 100 people and warned them that the side effects of the pill might include dizziness, nausea, and diarrhea, some of the subjects would actually develop those symptoms. The side effects would occur because emotions such as anxiety or depression, whatever would signal the body, through the pathways described above, that such effects were forthcoming.

"Aha," my psychiatrist friend might say, "that just proves that all diseases do originate in the mind, and that the mind can cure all diseases. What do you say to that?" I would say, "Well now, I just don't think that it proves any such thing, but I do think it shows that we have a vast new territory to explore. I think it shows that we probably have here a powerful mechanism for maintaining our health, enhancing our well-being, and increasing our longevity. I think it shows that we shouldn't send 'I give up' messages to our subconscious mind—and thus to our whole body—by constantly saying and/or thinking 'I'm getting sick,' or 'I'm getting old.'"

Can mental attitude and the way we approach life keep us young?

Some people who are 60 years old look like they are 40, and some people who are 40 years old look like they are 60. Some people are young at the age of 95 and some are old at the age of 55. I am convinced that two of the major factors responsible for these differences are the way individuals approach life in general and the way they approach day-to-day living in particular. I can't cite a major scientific study to support this belief, but there is ample evidence to show that emotions (and thought patterns) such as joy, ecstasy, happiness, anger, hostility, and depression influence the function, health, and well-being of the entire body. Although I can't cite specific findings to support the hypothesis that a person's state of mind is a major factor in prolonging his youth, I would like to give you my reasons for believing that it is.

People who are perpetually young seem to be preoccupied with the present moment. They are too busy with the here and now to search out, and dwell upon, all of the past and present tragedies in the universe. They accept the fact that change is one of the few certainties in life.

When they and the people and things around them change, they just accept those changes as evidence that the universe is still functioning as it should. It never occurs to them to send an "I'm getting old" message to their subconscious minds just because things look a little different today from the way they did yesterday.

People who are perpetually young seem to be content to allow life to "happen" naturally—to let it happen as it will, being neither offended nor feeling rejected if it happens a certain way. They are too busy with their own present moments to get frustrated because people and things don't function in the particular way they may expect. In fact, they don't have a lot of "shoulds" with regard to the way people do things. Their contentment seems to come from within and to be independent of external circumstances. They know that a traffic jam isn't capable of being concerned about what they think or feel and that it isn't going to go away just because they want it to. Since what's going on outside of them—traffic jams, political situations, or the actions of others—isn't concerned about what they think or feel, *they don't let such external things determine whether or not they are happy.* This attitude reduces wear and tear on their bodies and minds. People who are perpetually young can be serious about an occupation or hobby but can appreciate the value of a sense of humor.

How can having a sense of humor help?

A sense of humor seems to make some situations which would be unmanageable and unpalatable to the average person more manageable and more palatable to them. They seem to know that what they feel on the inside is determined by the way they think. Consequently, they choose—either instinctively or through learned behavior—to influence their emotions by the way they think. They choose to have a sense of humor, to laugh, to be happy. They are able to maintain a sense of humor because they don't constantly tell themselves that the world around them should be any way other than the way it is. Their sense of humor helps to keep them from getting mentally or physically old and probably helps to prevent emotional stagnation. A sense of humor sends an "I'm young and full of life" message to the body.

People who are perpetually young don't seem to react to the cry of alarmists. When they hear "bad" news, they automatically put it in perspective. When they hear the "bad" news that people are having problems because the weather is hot, cold, wet, or dry, they realize that during the course of any given year the weather is *always* hot, cold, wet, or dry, and that it will always be that way. When they hear the "bad" news that the Democrats/Republicans have been elected, they realize that the country has moved forward during the administrations of both Democrats and Republicans. When they hear the "bad" news about the economy, they realize that people are still buying cars, VCRs, video cameras, boats, bikes, and other "toys," that more money than ever before is being spent on sporting events, and that all of those new restaurants are opening up because more people are eating out than ever before. When they hear the "bad" news about our system of medical care, our poor nutrition, or our lack of physical fitness, they remind themselves of the dramatic increase in life expectancy during the past two decades.

The perpetually young seem to know that often news is news *only* if it is "bad." They seem to be able to accept the fact that whatever is, just *is;* that the terms "good" or "bad" might not necessarily apply. They don't put themselves through an episode of undue stress over something that just *is.* An oil shortage might be "bad" news to some (higher prices), and an oil glut might be "bad" news to others (fewer people employed). To the perpetually young, an oil shortage or an oil glut is something that just *is.* We could learn a lot from them.

Are we affected by how we perceive and analyze things?

Often the way we perceive and analyze an event does more to determine the amount of stress that it causes us than does the event itself. When problems or unexpected situations arise, the amount of stress to which we are subjected may be determined by the way we handle them rather than by the problems and situations themselves.

It just doesn't work to try to formulate an equation that says that a given stressor produces a given dysfunction. When two people are subjected to the same stressor, more often than not they will react to it differently. Something that is a stressor for one individual isn't a stressor for another. People who are perpetually young have learned that their brains, which have evolved over a period of some 500 million years, can attenuate either physical or psychological trauma. They have 100 *billion* brain cells to help them cope with virtually any situation that arises.

Summary

I am convinced that one's state of mind is vitally important in prolonging youth. Beliefs and attitudes produce measurable changes in the hormone levels in our body, and produce measurable changes in our immune system (and in the other systems of our body). These changes affect the rate at which we age.

Our ultimate biological limits are well beyond the century mark. A baby who is one year old today could live to be 120 years old. When she (or he) is 55 years old, she is probably going to look as young as today's 40-year-olds. When she is 85 years old, she will likely have the energy that the 65-year-olds of today have.

She certainly won't get into a rut when she is 50 or 60 years of age. She won't put a shawl over her shoulders and sit around talking to others who also have shawls over their shoulders. She will try new hair styles, new recipes, and new clothes. She will seek new experiences, travel to new places, and accept new challenges. She will be enthusiastic about life, not bored with it; she will be mentally active, not mentally lazy; she will be receptive to new ideas. She won't have hang-ups about things that she "can't" do, or that she "shouldn't" do at a certain age. She will have discovered the key to thinking young.

If we are going to test our biological limits, we must realize that our *belief* about our health, youthfulness, and longevity is important. Our attitude toward life in general, plus the way we approach day-to-day living, is important. I am certain that people in our society who are 60 years old but who look 40, and people who are young at the age of 95, have beliefs and attitudes that help them look and feel that way.

CHAPTER 10

Beauty is at Least Skin Deep

Isn't it gratifying that the entertainment industry has finally discovered that some of the most beautiful women in the world are over 40? Jacqueline Bisset, Catherine Deneuve, and Linda Evans are among them. There are millions of others who are every bit as beautiful. They just happen not to be as well known. Luck probably has very little to do with the way these women look. They simply do some things that other women don't do.

Turning back the aging clock requires a planned, all-out attack on *all* of the processes which cause premature aging. One of the organs of the body which must receive special attention, if one is to look young, is the skin, as well as the hair and nails which are skin appendages.

The skin is more than a covering. It is a remarkable organ. If you weigh 130 pounds, approximately 19 pounds (about 15 percent) of that weight is skin. The skin isn't just an inert covering stretched over the body. It has several very important functions. It protects the body against mechanical injury, chemical injury, and infectious agents. It protects against fluid loss. It is a barrier between the internal environment and the external one. The skin is a receptor for the sensations of heat, cold, touch, and pain, and, as such, provides information about the external environment.

A healthy, efficiently functioning skin is essential for proper body temperature regulation. If the body temperature begins to rise, the cooling effect of perspiration lowers it. If the body temperature tends to fall, blood vessels in the skin constrict and send the warm blood from the skin deeper toward the core of the body.

How does the skin function?

The skin consists of two main layers: the epidermis and the dermis.

The outside, or surface, layer is the epidermis. There is a constant turn-over of cells in this layer. As cells are lost from the epidermis, they are replaced. It's estimated that the entire epidermis is replaced approximately every 45 days.

The skin is metabolically active. It is a dynamic, living, functioning organ, just as much as the liver or any other organ of the body is. The skin contains cells (melanocytes) which produce pigment for protection against ultraviolet radiation and cells which function to prevent contact allergy.

Beneath the surface is a layer called the dermis. The dermis contains connective tissue, nerves, blood vessels, lymphatic vessels, sweat glands, oil-producing (sebaceous) glands, and hair follicles.

The skin and its associated structures—the hair, nails, and glands—are constantly changing. One of the most obvious manifestations of aging in the human body is the change in the skin. That means that if one uses a common sense approach to caring for the skin, it is possible for that person to look much younger than his or her chronological age. And many people, in the process of caring for their entire body, do take very good care of their skin.

I have a friend in her 40s whose vocation is exercising. She is a certified aerobics instructor who conducts one or two exercise classes a day, six days a week. Her well-conditioned muscles are a near-perfect example of strength, flexibility, and tone. Her skin appears to be just as healthy as her muscles. Most college-age women would probably be delighted if their skin and muscles were as healthy.

What do people who have young, healthy skin have in common?

I'll tell you what they do *not* have in common first. Not face-lifts, not facial collagen injections, not megavitamins, not quack food supplements, and not fad diets for weight control. Here's what they do have in common: (1) *They eat a well-balanced, low-fat diet;* (2) *they avoid undue exposure to the sun;* and (3) *they have a regular exercise program.*

Why is diet important for healthy skin?

A well-balanced, low-fat diet is important for several reasons. A primary reason is that it can help a person stay slim and energetic, which helps to keep *all* of the body systems, including the skin, young. Obesity ages the skin as well as the rest of the body. Obese people tend to have sagging faces. They develop jowls and double chins early. The other side of that coin is that a *rapid* weight loss causes the skin to lose some of its natural elasticity. When that happens, permanent wrinkles appear. Also, if the person doesn't lose the weight by about the age of 35, the wrinkles might appear (and be permanent) anyway.

A well-balanced diet helps keep the skin young in other ways. When a person is exposed to radiation, pollution, rancid fats, and other harmful agents, molecules called free radicals are formed. (Some free radicals are formed as normal day-to-day metabolic processes take place.) The free radicals flail about inside and outside the cells of the body destroying the cells and aging the body. There are several free radical "scavengers," or neutralizers of free radicals.

Can vitamins help my skin?

Two of the fat-soluble vitamins, vitamins A and E, and a water-soluble vitamin, vitamin C, help neutralize the effects of the free radicals. The element selenium is also a free radical scavenger. The inclusion of whole grains, fresh fruits, fresh vegetables, and seafood in one's diet will provide the vitamins and the selenium necessary to help neutralize the free radicals. Also, there is a red carotenoid pigment called lycopene in tomatoes and red fruits which neutralizes free radicals. To a lesser extent, the amino acid, cysteine, and the naturally occurring essential amino acid, methionine, are free radical scavengers.

How do fats and oils in the diet affect the skin?

Diets which are too low in fat, especially the essential fatty acids, cause the skin to assume an old, lifeless appearance. The essential fatty acids are linoleic and linolenic acids (see Chapter Four). A well-balanced diet contains a sufficient quantity of both. In fact, essential fatty acid deficiency is rare, except in cases of severe malnutrition, or in rare instances where individuals eat nothing but uncooked fruits and vegetables. As long as a minimum of 10 percent of the total calories in the diet comes from fat, developing an essential fatty acid deficiency is highly improbable.

What about Omega-3 and where are these oils found?

In addition to the essential fatty acids, the Omega-3 oils are important. Animals which are fed Omega-3 oils survive longer than those animals on a standard diet. Animals totally deprived of the Omega-3 oils show the characteristic signs of accelerated aging. These oils are found in cold-water fish and in food-grade linseed oil. The linseed oil may be the best source of the Omega-3, but there is another reason for eating fish.

Fish oils may also inhibit autoimmune diseases such as lupus and arthritis (*Americal Journal of Pathology*, April, 1987). Mice with lupus which received the fish oils—in contrast to animals which received diets containing equal amounts of fat in the form of lard or corn oil—had a reduced inflammation and death rate. This is an indication that the fish oils strengthen the immune system.

What goes on beneath the surface layer of skin?

It would seem that if all of the cells in the skin are replaced approximately every 45 days, the skin should have an eternally youthful appearance. It probably would have, except that much of the aging of the skin takes place beneath the surface layer (epidermis).

There are fibers of connective tissue in the skin which are made of protein. There are also elastic fibers in the skin. If the skin does not receive the proper care, both types of fibers fray and break. When that happens, wrinkles begin to appear. The effect usually isn't noticeable until after the age of 40. There are cells in the skin, called fibroblasts, which produce connective tissue fibers to replace the broken ones. The number of fibroblasts decreases with age. Consequently, the connective tissue fibers can't be as efficiently replaced.

There are two other changes in the skin which occur with age: the oil glands of the skin atrophy, and there is some pigmentation of the skin.

What does the sun do to our skin?

Excessive exposure to the sun accelerates all of these so-called age-related changes. (*Actually, the changes in the skin may be more related to diet, exposure to the sun, and exercise than to age.*)

Some experts say that as much as 70 percent of the so-called age-related changes in the skin is damage caused by the sun. The sun is particularly devastating to fair-skinned people, but it does damage, to a lesser extent, darker-skinned individuals. For older people, sitting in the sun is even more harmful. With age there is a decrease in the number of the pigment-containing cells in the skin.

Lotions which contain para-aminobenzoic acid (PABA) block the sun's harmful ultraviolet rays. These sunscreen lotions have numerical values indicating the degree of protection; the higher the number, the greater the protection offered. The Cancer Foundation recommends a screen with a protecton factor of at least 15 for people who are exposed to the sun. There are some newer sunscreens with protection factors much higher than 15. If a person is unable to avoid the sun, or if he chooses to play in the sun (I do because I like sailboats), he might remember to provide protection for his skin. The single most important thing that a person can do to prevent premature aging of the skin is *avoid the sun*.

Do moisturizers inhibit or reverse wrinkles?

Unfortunately, no. The most obvious effect of aging on the skin is wrinkle formation. Preventive maintenance will go a long way toward inhibiting wrinkle formation. Since we haven't always known about effective preventive maintenance, an entire industry has come into existence. Millions of dollars are spent each year on products which promotors promise will make the skin eternally youthful. Most of these products are moisturizers. All moisturizers, whether they cost $2 a quart or $130 an ounce, work exactly the same way: they trap moisture in the skin causing the skin cells to swell and temporarily fill some of the skin crevices. Moisturizers are useful skin-care products, but they neither inhibit nor reverse age-related skin changes.

Isn't there a new "miracle cure" for wrinkles?

I'm hesitant to call it a miracle cure, but the compound tretinoin—brand name Retin-A—does inhibit wrinkle formation and smooth out existing wrinkles by increasing the rate of cell turnover in the skin. The additional cells fill the crevices in the skin, thereby smoothing out the wrinkles. Retin-A promotes the production of new collagen in the skin, fades pigmented spots, and enhances the growth of new blood vessels, which improves the circulation in the skin. People with sun-damaged skin can benefit from the use of Retin-A.

Originally developed as an anti-acne agent, Retin A comes as a topical cream, gel, or lotion. It is absorbed into the body. Small quantities appear in the urine following topical application. The side effects of Retin-A use, when they do occur, appear to be minimal, consisting of symptoms such as flushing and itching. Obviously Retin-A is not recommended for use if a person has skin conditions such as eczema or sunburn. It is *essential* that users of Retin-A wear a sunscreen when outdoors because the skin's protective layer is thinned, making the skin more vulnerable to sun damage.

How can exercise prolong the youthfulness of the skin?

Exercise can prolong the youthfulness of the skin in several ways. It increases the deposition of collagen fibers and elastic fibers in the skin, which is essential since skin ages when these fibers start to disappear. Abundant quantities of elastic fibers and collagen fibers are the difference between young skin and old skin. Also, the sweating that results from exercise promotes an increased flow of nutrients to the skin and enhances the removal of metabolic waste products from it. This helps to keep the skin young.

Is sweating good for our skin?

Yes. Sweat glands are located in the outer layer of the skin. Ducts from the sweat glands transport perspiration to the surface of the skin. When the sweat evaporates, it cools the skin. During exercise an individual might lose several pints of fluid by perspiring.

There are small capillaries close to the surface of the skin. As blood flows through the capillaries, fluid containing vitamins, minerals, and nutrients filters out and flows to the sweat glands, bathing all the structures in the skin. These nutrients are not lost in the sweat, but stay in that bathing fluid.

If a person loses several pints of water by sweating, then an equal amount of fresh, nutrient-rich fluid must circulate in the spaces in the skin. The collagen fibers, elastic fibers, hair follicles, sebaceous glands, nerves, and lymphatic vessels are all bathed with this fresh fluid from the capillaries. This keeps those structures healthy as well as flushing out waste products. As people get older, they are (supposedly) not able to perspire as much as they did when they were young. With age, the sweat glands begin drying up. That is likely a result of disuse, not age. Continued exercise as a person ages will prolong the function of the sweat glands.

Exercise helps the skin to move, stretch, and rebound. That serves to strengthen the connective tissue components of the skin, just as exercise strengthens other parts of the body. When these components are strengthened, the skin looks younger.

It's little wonder that my friend who is an aerobics instructor has skin that looks young. Actually, the skin is *supposed* to look young. It's neglect that ages it.

Does nutrition affect our hair and nails?

Yes. Hair and nails, the skin's appendages, become healthier as the skin does.

The nails are plates of tightly packed keratinized cells. (Keratin is an insoluble fibrous protein.) Nails are constantly being replaced. Cell division takes place at the base of the nail. The white semicircular area there is a part of the area where this division takes place. The same good nutrition habits that make the skin healthy also make the nails healthy.

People who are in their early 20s are said to have the healthiest, best-looking hair. Older people's hair supposedly becomes thinner (especially men's hair) and loses some of its luster; however, this is not necessarily true. Hair grows to a certain length, enters a resting phase, and periodically sheds. The hair root is made of cells which continually divide to form the hair. Good, healthy skin enhances the health of the hair, although it does not necessarily prevent hair loss.

Does hair loss have to do with nutrition, too?

One of the causes of hair loss *is* poor nutrition. Hair is made of protein, and if there isn't sufficient protein in the diet, the growth and health of the hair will be compromised. Unnecessary hair loss will result and the hair which does remain will assume a duller appearance. Although, as we have seen, only 15 percent of one's calories need come from protein, the essential amino acids are absolutely necessary.

Other causes of hair loss include drugs such as antibiotics and certain tranquilizers, megavitamins (especially vitamin A), and imbalances such as insufficient thyroid hormone. On the other hand, shampooing the hair may thicken it. There is a substance in scalp oils which inhibits hair growth. Frequent shampooing can remove that substance and make the hair thicker.

Is there a way to prevent hair loss?

Thinning of the hair may be, of course, an inherited trait. That means that some people will lose their hair no matter what they do. But the hair that they do keep can be healthy. Now there is help for some people with inherited hair loss. There is a new drug called monoxidil (brand name Rogaine) which will promote hair growth. Apparently, if dormant hair follicles are present, Rogaine can stimulate them to be more active. This is a prescription drug, so a physician must be consulted.

NOTE: Quacks perform hair analysis to diagnose nonexistent conditions such as selenium poisoning or lead poisoning. Lead acetate is the active ingredient in anti-graying agents, and selenium is the active ingredient in dandruff-removing shampoos. Consequently, selenium and/or lead may be found when a hair analysis is done. Vitamin and mineral content of the body can be determined by analyzing living tissue, not hair. Quacks do hair analysis so they can sell lucrative supplements to individuals who are anxious about losing their hair.

Summary

To have young, healthy skin:

1. *Eat a well-balanced, low-fat diet.*
2. *Avoid undue exposure to the sun.*
3. *Exercise daily.*

Much new information about the skin is forthcoming. We will soon know more about how to maintain the youth and vitality of the skin.

Research is now being done on skin imaging. Measurement of skin thickness using ultrasound has been found to be concise and accurate. Ultrasound can be used repetitively on a particular skin area to determine changes due to disease processes or changes due to treatment.

The physical, mechanical, optical, and thermal properties as well as the physical basis for skin sensations are all being studied as are the structure, organization, and function of the large molecules in the skin. Even though it is now possible to significantly inhibit premature aging of the skin, all of this new information will make it even easier to do so.

It isn't surprising that the entertainment industry has discovered that some of the most beautiful women in the world are over 40. The discovery is long overdue.

CHAPTER 11

Muscle Strength and Flexibility are Here to Stay

When I was a youngster, several of my classmates and I, as many young people do, wanted to become good athletes. We often wondered what it took to build large muscles. One day a college athlete—a lineman on a championship football team—said to me, "Red meat builds muscle." I accepted the statement as fact. It was not until many years later that I learned that this concept, which many still believe to be true, is a complete myth.

Isn't red meat the best muscle builder?

Red meat doesn't build muscle any more than any other food. The complex carbohydrates are the best muscle-building foods. The beautiful Clydesdale horses which appear on the TV commercials are prime examples. They have massive amounts of muscle and they eat vegetables and grains.

There are other myths regarding the muscular system which need to be debunked. We have, for a long time, had some false notions about what happens to muscles as we grow older. Once we dispense with the myths, we can take a rational approach to caring for our muscular system. Physiologists tell us that, beginning at about the age of 30 in many people, there is a progressive loss of skeletal muscle which is replaced by fat. This loss of muscle is accompanied by a decrease in strength of contraction and speed of muscle reflexes. (Keep in mind that this is what happens to the *average* person.) But a large portion of the loss of muscle mass and strength is due to inactivity, not age. Age-related changes are not the reason that the average adult has trouble doing one pushup. The real cause is *disuse*.

What is muscle anyway?

There are three types of muscles in the human body. *Skeletal muscle,* named for its location, is attached to the bones and is a voluntary muscle. One can contract or relax skeletal muscle at will. *Cardiac muscle* forms the bulk of the wall of the heart and is an involuntary muscle. *Smooth muscle* is located in the walls of hollow structures such as blood vessels, intestines, trachea, and the ducts of glands. It is also involuntary.

All of the muscles of the body have one thing in common: they contract. Contraction usually produces movement. When skeletal muscles contract, the head, trunk, or limbs move. (Contraction of the skeletal muscles does not *always* produce movement. Muscles of the trunk may contract and maintain a state of tension to provide posture.) When cardiac muscle contracts, it propels blood through the vascular system. When smooth muscle contracts, it propels the contents of hollow structures, such as the intestine, along that structure.

A view through an electron microscope reveals that muscles have large filaments (myosin) and small filaments (actin) which are arranged in parallel rows. When muscles contract, or shorten, these filaments slide upon each other: the contraction produces movement. The energy for contraction comes from the compound adenosine triphosphate, or ATP. The muscles must have glycogen in order to produce ATP.

What happens when a muscle meets resistance?

When a muscle is exercised against a resistance (i.e. the lifting of a weight), the size of the muscle increases. This is called hypertrophy. The diameter of the individual muscle cells increases due to the gain in total quantity of contractile elements. There are a number of little "power houses," called mitochondria, in the muscle cells. Energy for muscle contraction is generated in these power houses. When a muscle is exercised, there is an increase in the number of these energy-producing components.

Exercise will stimulate the muscle cells to store extra nutrients such as glycogen. Thus muscular hypertrophy increases both the structural components of the muscle (which will give it increased power) and the nutrients necessary for producing that power.

Exercise can build strength and flexibility only in the muscles of the young, right?

Wrong! Almost anyone who is in good general health can train his or her muscles to store enough energy to allow for running a marathon.

There are thousands of people, men and women, over the age of 60 who are doing that very thing. Noel K. Johnson, for instance, was 70 years old, 50 pounds overweight, and in bad shape. Instead of entering a nursing home, as his son suggested, he began an exercise program, gradually increased his strength and endurance, and eventually was able to spend three hours a day running, trampolining, and weight lifting. By the time he had reached the age of 88, he had run six New York City Marathons. (*Business Week*, February 8, 1988, McGraw Hill Co.)

Can older people ever be strong again?

It's another myth that older people can't respond to strength training. They can. We have long had anecdotal evidence of this, and now we have scientific evidence.

The well-designed study (*Journal of Applied Physiology*, March, 1988) gave clear evidence that strength training resulted in a *"remarkable increase in muscle strength and size"* in older people (italics mine). Since it was previously believed that older people *couldn't* respond to weight training, they weren't challenged to try very hard to increase their muscle strength and size. Obviously, since they weren't challenged, they didn't see much gain. The participants in the study who were challenged benefited from the exercise. According to the author, "The men in the study greatly improved their functional capacity because they gained strength."

Can older people "handle the heat?"

Another myth which has now been eliminated is that older people can't train themselves to handle the heat which is produced during exercise. Heat is produced when muscles contract and remain in a state of contraction. When a young person exercises regularly, his body learns to cope more efficiently with the increased heat production. It has now been shown that this works exactly the same way in an older person. Endurance training or aerobic fitness such as that gained from walking, jogging, biking, or swimming helps older individuals cope with the heat produced during exercise. In fact, young sedentary men (average age 21 years) were *less* able to exercise in heat than physically fit middle-aged men (average age 46 years). The middle-aged men who had been training for several years were able to walk for a two-hour period; they sweated more profusely; and they maintained a lower core and skin temperature than the younger men, who became exhausted 27 minutes earlier (*Journal of Applied Physiology* 65(1):65-71, 1988).

If exercise is so good, why doesn't everybody do it?

Even though we can increase our strength and flexibility by exercising, many of us simply don't do it. We have all kinds of excuses. People say, "As soon as I get a little stronger, I'm going to start exercising." That's like saying, "As soon as this cold room warms up some, I'm going to turn on some heat." One must first exercise in order to gain strength.

Other individuals claim that they are reluctant to engage in exercises which might increase the size of their muscles because they fear it will hamper their flexibility. That is a myth. Stretching exercises increase flexibility, and it is the lack of stretching exercises, not muscular development, that inhibits flexibility. Women can use weight training to increase both strength and endurance without building bulky muscles because they have a lower level of a hormone (testosterone) which promotes muscular hypertrophy.

Will lifting weights hurt my heart?

I have heard people say, "If I work out with weights, even light weights, to tone up my muscles, it might cause me to have an 'enlarged heart.'" That is also a myth, although it remains a common belief. Both running and weight lifting do cause the heart to increase in size which allows it to pump more blood with each beat and to beat fewer times each minute. Previously, exercise physiologists thought that weight lifting caused an increase in the thickness of the wall of the heart, but not an increase in the size of the cavity.

The research of Jean G. Dumesnil has shown that this is not the case. His research team found that weight lifters' hearts increase in wall thickness *and* cavity size (*Journal of Applied Physiology* 64:2552-2557, 1988). Most health professionals believe that running and other aerobic exercises do more for the heart than bodybuilding, but both running and weight lifting strengthen the heart.

I am not trying to persuade you to engage in heavy exercise so that you can accumulate huge, bulky masses of muscle. I am citing evidence which shows that forced muscle activity does not harm the heart, and that it can go a long way toward preventing the reduction in muscle mass often erroneously attributed to aging. (In the previous chapter we discussed the sagging skin that is sometimes seen in older people. This may not be sagging skin so much as a decrease in muscle tone and size.)

Is it possible to exercise more efficiently?

We might soon be able to exercise more efficiently in order to maintain good muscle tone and muscle mass. During exercise, animals—humans included—have to metabolize glycogen, produce ATP, and contract their muscles. Oxygen is required to metabolize, or burn, glycogen. If a person sprints for a short distance, he uses oxygen faster than he can breathe it into his body. After he stops running, he must breathe hard for a few minutes to pay back the oxygen that he used. Some animals are better at that than others.

Thoroughbred horses can continue running even when their bodies are very low on oxygen (*Journal of Applied Physiology*, February, 1988). The horses can build up an oxygen debt two to three times what humans can develop. By studying animals with different capacities for exercise, scientists hope to find the factors which limit exercise ability in humans. This might enable humans to perform more efficient exercises in order to maintain their muscle mass and tone.

What role does nutrition play in muscle building?

Proper nutrition is vitally important in inhibiting the loss of muscle tissue with age. Complex carbohydrate in the diet is required to provide the body with glucose—the body's basic energy source. If the body is not getting enough complex carbohydrate in the diet, it will attempt to obtain the glucose from stored fat. If a lot of calories are required, the fatty acids will be incompletely broken down, forcing the body to obtain the glucose from other sources. Unfortunately, the other sources are the muscles and the major body organs, such as the heart. Thus, an attempt to increase muscle tone and size while following an improper diet can actually result in a *decrease* in the size of the muscles. The message here is that daily exercise of the different muscle groups *plus* a diet which ensures an adequate intake of carbohydrates will prevent undue muscle loss with age.

Does maintaining muscle mass increase life expectancy?

Not necessarily, but exercise is required to maintain muscle mass, and exercise *does* increase one's life expectancy. Maintaining muscle mass and tone will help to keep you looking younger. You could lose a great deal of muscle mass and still live to be 110 years of age. But wouldn't you rather live to be 110 years of age and, at the same time, have a greatly improved functional capacity because of your muscle flexibility and strength?

Exercise is about 50 percent mental and 50 percent physical. About half of the total effort of exercising is the mental effort required to get started. Think of it this way: once you *begin* to exercise, the job is half-finished. There are a multitude of rewards for exercising, not the least of which is a young muscular system...no matter what your chronological age.

Summary

You can build and maintain muscle strength and flexibility with regular exercise and proper diet.

And you'll feel terrific doing it!

CHAPTER 12

Breathe New Life Into Your System

We have been misled again. We have been told that as we reach the age of 30 or so, the amount of air that we can breathe into our lungs decreases approximately eight to ten percent with each passing decade. We have been told that the six quarts of air we are able to breathe into our lungs when we are 30 years old will dwindle to a mere three quarts by the time we are 70. Well, guess what? This decline in respiratory function is not primarily an effect of aging.

If aging isn't the primary cause of respiratory changes in our system, what is?

Some recent studies have shown that these changes, like so many other "age-related" changes, are primarily a result of *disuse*, not aging. The effect of exercise is so pronounced that just one or two hours of exercise a week will dramatically slow this decline in respiratory function. If the cells of the body are to remain young and functional, every single cell must have a continuous supply of oxygen. Blood may flow freely through the blood vessels to the cells, but if that blood doesn't have a rich supply of oxygen, the function of the cells will be compromised. Since all of the cells of the body require oxygen, oxygen affects every aspect of a person's looks.

Visualize a cell deep within your body. Now visualize a molecule of oxygen floating around in the air. Can the two get together? Well, unless that molecule of oxygen can reach that cell, the cell cannot continue to function. They do get together by the process known as respiration. Respiration is an all-inclusive term which means that oxygen is transported from the air to the cells of the body, and that carbon dioxide is transported from the cells of the body back into the air. Respiration includes several steps and involves more than just the movement of air in and out of the lungs, although that is an essential part of it.

144

The term "VO2 max" is an abbreviation for maximum oxygen utilization. It is a general measure of how efficiently the body can use oxygen. The efficiency with which the body can use oxygen depends on the efficiency of respiration.

What are the requirements for efficient respiration?

There are several requirements: (1) There must be an inflow and outflow of air between the atmosphere and the alveoli (the small air sacs deep within the lungs). (2) Oxygen must diffuse from the alveoli into the blood, and carbon dioxide must diffuse from the blood into the alveoli. (3) Oxygen must be carried by the red blood cells to the tiny capillaries which are near the cells of the body. There the oxygen diffuses from the red blood cells into the cells of the body. Carbon dioxide diffuses from the cells of the body into the red blood cells, and is transported back to the lungs. (4) The body must be able to regulate the rate of respiration so that adequate oxygen is supplied to the cells of the body and the carbon dioxide is removed.

A breakdown in any of the above four steps will result in a cessation of respiration—that molecule of oxygen that you visualized in the air will not be able to reach that single cell deep inside your body.

Do the lungs deserve equal billing with the heart?

Much emphasis is placed on preventing heart disease so that a person may have a longer, healthier life, and that's as it should be, but the respiratory system should receive equal billing. If respiration ceases, the cells of the body will die very quickly. If the function of the respiratory system is compromised, the function of some of the cells of the body may be compromised within a matter of minutes. We must exercise and protect our respiratory system if we want it to remain robust until the end of our 110-year life span.

The diaphragm, the large muscle beneath the rib cage, contracts to pull air into the lungs. It does this in a rhythmical fashion during normal quiet breathing and more vigorously during a very deep inspiration. During a deep inspiration, the muscles of the rib cage also contract, raising the rib cage and pulling additional air into the lungs.

What can we do to keep our lungs from weakening?

We must breathe deeply and frequently. If you take as deep a breath as possible and then exhale all of the air that you possibly can, that volume of air is called the *vital capacity*. The average adult's vital capacity is five to six quarts. As we get older, or so we are told, the vital capacity decreases. This happens because the diaphragm and other muscles of respiration weaken; because the ligaments and other tissues in the chest stiffen; and because the lungs can't expand as well as they once could. We *allow* most of these changes to take place. When they do, the amount of air that we can breathe into and out of our lungs is reduced.

Why do we "allow" age-related changes? Can we prevent them?

A deep breath will require more effort, and it won't be as deep as it once was. The degree to which these changes occur depends on the steps we take to prevent premature aging of the respiratory system. Maybe we aren't *supposed* to be able to prevent these "age-related" changes, but we can. Besides, how can we be good at doing anything unless we think we can do something that we're not supposed to be able to do in the first place? I learned a little about this from a runner who is 20 years older than I am.

After being in school for a period of time and then spending several years getting a career underway, I was "out of shape" because I had not exercised properly. (Being in school and working are excuses, not reasons for not exercising.) Once I began exercising again, I felt really good. I decided to enter a 5-kilometer (3.1-mile) road race. One of the runners was 20 years my senior, and I thought that he would insure that I didn't finish last.

As it turned out, I wasn't the last person to finish, but when I crossed the line, I found that he had already finished the race, cooled down, put on his warm-ups, and was cheering other runners like me across the line. I wondered how that could be. His VO2 max—maximum oxygen consumption—was supposed to have declined over the years to a level that was some 15 to 20 percent below mine. If that were so, how could he outrun me? I figured out pretty quickly that the changes that are *supposed* to take place in the respiratory system with age don't *necessarily* take place. I had been misled. Although the respiratory system of the *average* person does change as I had been taught, this particular runner just wasn't "average."

The muscles of his respiratory system and the flexibility of his chest cage had been maintained because he took very deep breaths during his periods of exercise. These deep breaths strengthened his diaphragm and the muscles of his chest wall. Once the clean, oxygenated air reached his lungs, the oxygen was easily transferred from the alveoli into the red blood cells since there was apparently no emphysema or other lung disease. As long as this man continues to exercise, he will probably have a healthy respiratory system.

We are told that, with age, some of the alveoli in the lungs rupture. When that happens, they are no longer useful in transferring oxygen into the blood. When many alveoli rupture, they merge to form large air sacs with a reduced overall volume and surface area for oxygen transfer; consequently, less oxygen can be transferred from the lungs into the blood. I don't believe that alveoli just spontaneously "rupture" as one gets older, or we would all have the same amount of emphysema.

What causes the air sacs in the lungs to rupture?

Here is one reason why alveoli rupture: within the tube that carries air to the lungs (the trachea) and the branches of the trachea (the bronchi) are cells which secrete mucus. These cells are called goblet cells. When smoke and other pollutants are inhaled, the goblet cells respond by secreting an excessive amount of mucus. This makes the cilia in the trachea and bronchi less effective. (Cilia are hairlike processes which project from the surface of the trachea and bronchi. They move foreign material out of the lungs and into the throat.) When the cilia are not effective, mucus is not carried toward the throat. It remains trapped in the bronchial tubes and collects in the air sacs. This causes millions of air sacs to rupture, reducing the diffusion surface for the transfer of oxygen into the blood.

If all of the air sacs in the lungs of a normal adult were opened up and flattened out, they would cover an area of approximately 600 square feet. That's equivalent to the floor area of a room that is 20 feet wide and 30 feet long. With such a large surface for the exchange of oxygen between the lungs and the blood, it's little wonder that the oxygen can pass so quickly from the lungs into the blood, or that carbon dioxide can pass so easily from the blood into the lungs. If we keep our alveoli healthy, large supplies of fresh oxygen can *always* pass from our lungs into our blood.

What damage does smoking do? And will quitting stop the injury?

When constant irritation by smoke and other pollutants destroys the alveoli, they are gone forever to be replaced with connective tissue. If we stop inhaling pollutants, that will prevent further damage to the alveoli, but the destroyed ones will never be restored. We are fooling ourselves if we say we are going to stop smoking "one day" so that our injured lungs can return to normal. We can stop the injury, but returning the lungs to normal is another matter.

We must come to grips with the things that will improve our health, *and do them*. We must be motivated out of a desire to get better and better. Our motivation won't last very long if it is only motivation to patch up things as they go wrong. We must be motivated to learn more and more about how to keep ourselves healthy.

How does oxygen reach all our tissues?

Let us assume that we have healthy alveoli, and that oxygen can easily pass from the alveoli into the red blood cells. The oxygen will reach all of the tissues of the body (1) if there are a sufficient number of red blood cells; (2) if those red blood cells contain hemoglobin; and (3) if the blood is flowing freely in the blood vessels. Let's examine each of those three "ifs" individually, beginning with the red blood cells.

The life span of the red blood cell is estimated to be 120 days, which means that all of the red blood cells in the body are replaced about every four months. This requires that the normal rate of red blood cell production be approximately 500 milliliters, or about one pint per month. If a person suffers blood loss, the body can produce red blood cells at approximately four times that rate. Vitamin B12 is essential if red blood cell production is to take place at a rate sufficient to replace those that are continually lost (see Chapter Six). While vitamin B12 (which is found in meat and dairy products) is necessary for red blood cell production, supplements or megadoses of the vitamin do not guarantee a better supply, or a better quality of red blood cells.

What makes the red blood cells functional?

If the red blood cells are to be functional, they must contain hemoglobin. Hemoglobin is the compound inside the red blood cells to which oxygen must bind so that it can be transported to the tissues of the body. An adequate supply of iron is necessary for hemoglobin formation (see Chapter Six). Since iron is found in green leafy vegetables, legumes, whole grains, and lean meat, iron supplements aren't necessary unless a hemoglobin deficiency has been demonstrated. Copper is another element which is required for hemoglobin production. Copper deficiency is rare, but it could occur in individuals who are too long on a fad diet. Copper deficiency inhibits the ability of the bone marrow to synthesize hemoglobin. Copper is found in seafood and fortified bran.

The third requirement is that the oxygenated blood must be able to flow freely through the blood vessels to the various tissues of the body. *As far as the tissues are concerned, the oxygen "ain't there 'til it's there."* I have discussed the importance of maintaining the health of the heart and blood vessels elsewhere in this book, but I will repeat this point: fat intake must be reduced so that the high fat levels in the blood don't cause the red blood cells to clump. If the red blood cells aren't stuck together, they can flow more easily through the blood vessels to the tissues of the body. When the blood reaches the tissues and flows through the tiny capillaries which are close to the individual cells of the body, the red blood cells will go through the capillaries single file. This means that the oxygen will more quickly diffuse from the red blood cells to the cells of the body.

Is breathing always automatic?

Yes. Although we can purposely inhale or exhale air, most of the time we breathe without being aware of it. The center which controls the respiratory rhythm is in the hypothalamus. An electrical impulse cycles in the hypothalamus and stimulates the inspiratory center to cause inspiration. A few seconds later it triggers the expiratory center to cause expiration. The cycle repeats itself over and over.

If a person needs to take deeper breaths and/or breathe faster, the respiratory center in the hypothalamus causes this to happen automatically, in a precisely controlled process. There are oxygen sensors in the blood vessels which send signals to the respiratory center. If the oxygen level in the blood begins to drop, the sensors signal the respiratory center to speed up the rate of respiration. If the level of carbon dioxide in the body begins to rise (because of increased physical exertion or for any other reason), sensors signal the respiratory center to speed up the rate of respiration to get rid of the extra carbon dioxide. The same oxygen and carbon dioxide sensors signal the respiratory center to slow the rate of respiration when required, as during sleep.

Anticipating strenuous exercise can cause the respiratory rate (and the heart rate) to increase. This happens when an athlete is on the starting line getting set to race. He begins to breathe faster and his heart starts to beat more rapidly, although he has not yet used any extra oxygen. The anticipation sets off a series of reactions that prepares the body for action.

The respiratory center in the brain which controls all these things operates perfectly for an entire lifetime unless it is injured. If a stroke or other disease severely injures an individual's respiratory center, that individual might not be able to survive.

Summary

Take an objective look at your respiratory system. People function at peak efficiency and feel the most energized when oxygen is being transported rapidly and freely to the cells of the body and carbon dioxide is being removed. If the respiratory system doesn't function for just a few minutes, the cells of the body—the brain cells first, and then the other cells—begin to die. The inhibition of the aging of the respiratory system must be a number one priority, and this can be accomplished by following some simple, straightforward steps.

Regular exercise is an absolute must. When a person exercises, the respiratory center in the brain forces that person to take the deepest breaths possible. In rare instances where people cannot exercise, they should purposely take deep breaths on a daily basis. That will help strengthen the respiratory muscles and maintain the flexibility of the rib cage.

Smoke and other pollutants must not be inhaled. They will paralyze the villi in the trachea and bronchi and will cause emphysema.

Some attention must be given to the diet. Foods which contain vitamin B12, iron, and copper will help make it possible for the body to have an adequate supply of healthy red blood cells so that oxygen can be transported into the body and carbon dioxide can be transported out.

As people get older, they can continue to efficiently use oxygen. The maximum oxygen consumption, or V02 max, doesn't have to decrease by approximately 10 percent with each passing decade. A good supply of oxygen affects just about every aspect of a person's looks: the skin, muscles, bone formation, and metabolism.

When you get your respiratory system in peak condition, don't assume that you can run—or walk, or swim, or bike—faster than someone else just because he or she happens to be 20 years older than you are. You might be in for a surprise.

CHAPTER 13

Getting to the Heart of the Matter

The beneficial effects of good nutrition and aerobic exercise on the cardiovascular system are discussed throughout this book. In this chapter we will look at specific age-related changes which occur in the cardiovascular system and examine steps which can be taken to inhibit those changes.

The resting heart of a 30-year-old man who weighs 150 pounds will pump approximately four quarts of blood per minute. (The amount of blood that the heart pumps in a given period of time is called the cardiac output.) By the time he reaches the age of 70, his cardiac output will have decreased. His resting heart will pump a little less than three quarts per minute. His heart doesn't pump less blood because it beats more slowly; his resting heart rate stays about the same. His heart pumps less blood with each beat because it has gotten weaker. Or at least this is what happens to the average person.

What causes the heart to get weaker as it ages?

A significant part of the decrease in cardiac output with age is caused by inactivity, not aging. Since the heart is a muscle and exercise maintains the vigor of muscles, exercise maintains the vigor of the heart. A lifetime program of aerobic exercise will blunt the reduction in resting cardiac output "caused" by aging.

The heart of a person of any age beats faster during exercise. At the age of 30, the maximum heart rate is approximately 200 beats per minute. By the age of 70 there has been a 25 percent reduction in the maximum heart rate during exercise—a reduction which, as you might guess, is not altogether age-related.

Isn't heart disease the leading cause of death?

Yes, but heart and blood vessel diseases do not *have* to be the most common cause of death in the United States. The lifestyle that a person chooses goes a long way toward determining his chances of having heart and blood vessel disease. The myth that the heart and the blood vessels in both men and women begin to become fragile as they age is debunked by the fact that many people in their 80s get out and run marathons.

What is a "normal" cardiovascular system?

The resting blood pressure of a 20-year-old is usually about 120/70. It will "normally" rise to about 150/85 by the time he reaches the age of 70 and will go higher if he develops hypertension. But a rise in blood pressure with age is not necessarily "normal." Inactivity and weight gain, both of which "normally" occur with age, are probably responsible for most of the increase in blood pressure.

A healthy 20-year-old who is eating a balanced diet may have a blood-cholesterol level of 180 milligrams per deciliter (mg/dl) or less. Since blood-cholesterol levels "normally" increase with age, his blood-cholesterol level might well be 20 percent higher by the time he is 70. Of course, if he continues to eat a balanced diet, doesn't gain weight, and remains active, his blood-cholesterol levels might not increase at all. This is yet another example of blaming the aging process for a change which is more likely brought on by a change in lifestyle.

There are approximately five million people in the United States who are 85 years old or older. Thousands of people live for more than 100 years. Does this not dramatically illustrate that, with proper care, the heart and blood vessels are capable of functioning in an efficient fashion for prolonged periods of time?

What if my cardiovascular system is damaged already?

It's likely that many of us already have some damaged blood vessels, the beginnings of atherosclerosis. We may not have eaten properly or taken care of our bodies in other ways when we were younger. There is nothing we can do about the past except learn from it. So let us begin taking better care of our hearts and our blood vessels *today*. There is some evidence that hardening of the arteries may now be reversible (see Chapter Five).

There are some effective, scientifically verified methods for prolonging the health of the heart and blood vessels. These methods are a direct result of an all-out assault on heart and blood vessel disease by such organizations as the National Institutes of Health and the American Heart

Association. By utilizing their research findings (and not the opinion of some layperson who decides to become a medical authority), we can do much to prevent heart and blood vessel disease. Let's pursue this a bit further.

Making sure that the lining on the inside of the blood vessels is not injured is extremely important. A minor occasional injury is not a problem; if the tissue is infrequently injured, it will heal just as would a scratch on the arm. The problem arises when there is repeated injury to the lining of a vessel, particularly an artery.

With repeated injury, the wall of the artery will start to thicken, and metabolic end-products as well as fat and calcium will accumulate in the thickened area of the wall. The result is hardening of the arteries, or atherosclerosis, which, if unchecked, will eventually block the artery. Two of the complications of atherosclerosis are heart attack and stroke. Also, if atherosclerosis occludes an artery which supplies an organ such as the kidney, that organ will become nonfunctional. These complications can be avoided by preventing atherosclerosis.

What causes atherosclerosis and what can we do to prevent it?

The causes of injury to the lining of the arteries are *high blood pressure*, *high blood levels of cholesterol*, and *toxic substances* such as carbon monoxide. Steps can be taken to prevent these injuries.

Maintaining a normal body weight and exercising on a regular basis will help greatly in maintaining a normal blood pressure. Diet, weight control, and exercise will help control blood-cholesterol levels. These factors also help promote a favorable balance in your blood of substances known as high-density lipoproteins (HDL) and low-density lipoproteins (LDL). The primary source of carbon monoxide is cigarette smoke, although automobile emissions and industrial pollutants may also contribute. The way to eliminate carbon monoxide from these sources is obvious.

If diet and exercise do not eliminate high blood pressure, medication may be required. High blood pressure should be brought under control not only because it injures the cells which line the inside of the arteries, but also because it causes the wall of the heart to thicken. Control of blood pressure is essential to good cardiovascular health. The level of blood pressure must be determined by measurement, not by the way a person feels. You may feel fine and still have high blood pressure.

How much cholesterol is too much?

Cardiovascular disease is not a rare disease which some people occasionally get. More than 2,000 people in the United States die of heart and blood vessel disease *every day*. Even moderately elevated levels of blood cholesterol can markedly increase the risk of dying from heart disease. *There is more than a two percent increase in mortality for each unit increase in blood cholesterol.* Men who are in the 35 to 57 age range and who have blood-cholesterol levels of 203 to 220 milligrams per deciliter (mg/dl) have death rates that are 73 percent higher than those whose blood-cholesterol levels are below 182 mg/dl. Men whose blood-cholesterol levels are above 245 mg/dl have death rates 242 percent higher than those whose blood-cholesterol levels are below 182 mg/dl.

How does cholesterol get into the blood?

The cholesterol in the blood comes from two sources: diet (it can be absorbed directly from the intestine into the blood without previous digestion) and the body's own production. Cholesterol itself is a useful compound. Its basic nucleus is used by the body as a building block to make hormones. *Excess* cholesterol is the problem.

Too much cholesterol or too many saturated fats in the diet will raise the blood-cholesterol levels, as will conditions such as diabetes or low amounts of thyroid hormone. The liver can manufacture cholesterol or take cholesterol out of the blood, depending upon the body's requirements. But if there is too much cholesterol in the blood for the liver to handle, the blood-cholesterol levels will remain high. Proper eating habits can go a long way toward lowering the blood-cholesterol levels in most individuals; this means reducing the amount of cholesterol, saturated fat, and total fat in the diet. Unfortunately, we all too often look for an easy way out.

Is there an easy way to reduce the blood-cholesterol level?

I was asked this not long ago on a talk radio show. One of the callers said that he had been told that almost everybody needed to lower their blood-cholesterol level to some degree. He wanted to know why scientists couldn't develop a pill that would produce this effect; then people could eat whatever they wanted and still have a low blood-cholesterol level. There are several things wrong with this line of reasoning.

First, cardiovascular fitness should, and does, come from good health practices, and not from a pill. Second, pills (and there are some on the market which will lower blood-cholesterol levels) are costly, and they would have to be taken forever. Third, judging from the way the average person takes prescribed medication, even if such pills were available and were free of charge, most people wouldn't take them on a regular basis.

A few individuals have a hereditary condition that causes them to have high blood-cholesterol levels which do not respond well to diets. These people can be treated with cholesterol-lowering drugs.

What about oat bran?

Oat bran, which is getting a lot of attention at present, is not a magic solution. Oat bran does bind with cholesterol, thereby helping to lower the blood-cholesterol levels. The problem is eating a sufficient amount of it every day. Eating some cereal every morning with a smattering of oat bran in it won't offset the harmful effects of bad eating habits. Include oat bran in your diet, it you like it, but don't consider it a cure-all for elevated blood-cholesterol levels.

What are HDLs and LDLs?

Substances in the blood called high-density lipoproteins protect against the development of atherosclerosis. Lipids (fats) in the blood which are attached to protein molecules are called lipoproteins. Some of these compounds are heavier—have a higher density—than others and they are called high-density lipoproteins (HDL). Those with the lower density are called low-density lipoproteins (LDL).

The exact mechanism by which high blood levels of the "good" HDL protects against atherosclerosis is not completely understood. Perhaps the HDL makes the cells lining the blood vessels stronger and more durable or protects them in some other fashion. If the HDL protects the lining cells from repeated injury, that would help prevent the development of atherosclerosis. The "bad" LDL speeds the development of atherosclerosis; perhaps by causing the cells lining the blood vessels to become weaker and more fragile. Another explanation is that HDL takes cholesterol out of the wall of blood vessels, while LDL adds cholesterol.

It's desirable to have high blood levels of the "good" HDL and low blood levels of the "bad" LDL in order to keep the cardiovascular system young and healthy. How can this be accomplished? Weight reduction (when it is necessary) and aerobic exercise both raise the level of HDL in the blood. The blood level of the harmful LDL can be lowered when there is less saturated fat, less total fat, and fewer cholesterol-containing foods in the diet.

What's the first step toward "cleaning up my heart"?

A total plan that includes several approaches to maintaining a healthy cardiovascular system is important. However, if you smoke, haven't exercised in 20 years, eat a diet that is 50 percent fat, have a blood-cholesterol level that is 300 mg/dl, and need to lose 30 pounds, by all means take that first step and do *something*. You needn't try to change everything at once. Begin by walking, then reduce the number of calories that you get from fat, and so on. One healthful activity will lead to another. But remember that you are aiming at an all-inclusive program in order to prevent premature aging of the cardiovascular system.

People have already begun practicing preventive medicine with respect to heart and blood vessel disease. As a result, they are living longer. The effectiveness of the programs is reflected in the decrease in mortality rates. Deaths from heart attacks fell by approximately 28 percent from 1976 to 1986 and deaths from stroke by approximately 40 percent during that same period (American Heart Association Annual Meeting, January 16, 1989). The declining death rates reflect better diets, more exercise, less smoking, and more effective treatment of high blood pressure. As more and more people accept and follow the known health practices for good cardiovascular health, the death rates will continue to decline.

What if I have a heart attack anyway?

People who do have heart attacks should seek treatment immediately. Of the people who have heart attacks, more than half die before reaching the hospital. But more than half of all victims wait longer than two hours before going to an emergency room. Early attention is vitally important, especially in view of the promising new drugs which have been developed to dissolve the blood clots that form in the narrowed arteries and block blood flow to the heart.

Do men have more heart attacks than women?

Sometimes we tend to think of heart disease as a man's disease, but heart disease is no respecter of sex. Almost a half million women—more than 1,200 per day—die each year of cardiovascular disease. The average risk of a heart attack for women who have reached their later 40s is about the same as for men.

A comprehensive 10-year study of 2,802 women has provided compelling evidence that it is important for women to exercise (Ekelund, 61st Scientific Sessions, American Heart Association, November 15, 1988). The study showed that *women who don't exercise are three times more likely to die of a heart attack than those who stay in shape.* The same study showed that 87 percent of women in their mid-40s don't have a program of regular exercise. Approximately 68 percent of men in the same age group don't have such a program. The fact that more men than women in their mid-40s exercise is probably a reflection of the belief that heart disease is primarily a man's problem. It isn't. In fact, according to Ekelund, women die from a first heart attack more often than do men.

Summary

Here are ways to improve the health of your heart and blood vessels and help them to function for a longer period of time:

1. *Check your blood-cholesterol level.* If it is too high, take steps to bring it below 180 mg/dl. You can do this by *permanently* reducing your intake of saturated fat, total fat (saturated or unsaturated), and cholesterol. If necessary, consult your physician about the possibility of taking Mevacor, niacin, or one of the other cholesterol-lowering drugs.

2. *Have your blood pressure measured.* If it is high, take whatever steps are necessary to bring it *all the way back back to normal*, whether that means lifestyle changes or taking medication.

3. *Eat some fresh fruit.* Your body needs potassium. There is evidence that a high intake of potassium can offer protection against stroke.

4. *Maintain a normal body weight.*

5. *Raise the level of the "good" HDL in your blood by exercising and losing excess weight.*

6. *Lower the level of the "bad" LDL in your blood by eating less saturated fat and fewer cholesterol-containing foods.*

7. *Stop smoking.* Scientists estimate that individuals who smoke throughout their adult lives decrease their life expectancy by eight years.

8. *Make exercise a part of your way of life.* Exercise will help prevent the "age-induced" decrease in cardiac output and will help keep the heartbeats from becoming weaker with age. Exercise will reduce the blood pressure, increase the blood HDL levels, reduce the resting heart rate, reduce the risk of heart attack, and increase the life expectancy.

9. *Eat the type of diet which has been advocated throughout this book.* Include copper to help your bone marrow synthesize hemoglobin; zinc (from seafood) so that the enzyme carbonic anhydrase can be formed in sufficient quantities to transport carbon dioxide out of your body; iron for hemoglobin formation; chromium so that a deficiency will not develop which would affect glucose tolerance and help raise the blood-cholesterol levels. Include folic acid (from oranges and/or spinach) in your diet so that your body can efficiently replace the millions of cells which are lost daily.

10. *Don't take megavitamins or mineral supplements* unless they have been prescribed by a physician for a demonstrated medical condition.

If all of this seems like too much to remember, try thinking of it this way: *Just eat a balanced diet and go take a hike!*

CHAPTER 14

You Can Digest Food
and Stand Straight
Even if You're Over 40

Mrs. Sarah Cannon, 76, keeps physically fit by playing tennis and walking. She chooses tennis partners who are better than she is so she can improve her game. She keeps her mind active with crossword puzzles. She is perky and full of life.

She radiates energy as she entertains, which she has been doing for nearly a half century on the Grand Ole Opry. Better known as Cousin Minnie Pearl, she has fans of all ages. Healthy, robust and active people such as Minnie Pearl are changing our ideas and attitudes about aging. They are a reflection of the way the current young generation is likely to be in years to come.

In future years we will be able to continue to do many things, including eating good food and standing up straight, because we will have a healthy digestive system and a strong skeletal system.

After a certain number of years have passed—after we get "old" (whatever that is)—we aren't going to have to sit around with a shawl over our shoulders, talk about the weather, and eat bland, strained food. Our digestive systems will change somewhat, but as with the other systems of the body, many of the changes can be prevented or slowed down. Often changes in the digestive system are due to disuse and abuse rather than age.

How does the aging process affect the digestive system?

Physiologists tell us that there are two things, in particular, about the digestive system that change with age. One is a decrease in the amount of the secretions necessary for digestion, and the other is a decrease in the muscular movement (motility) of the wall of the digestive system. These two basic changes lead to other problems with the digestive system such as indigestion, malabsorption, constipation, and gastritis.

People who are "old" but who seem to have healthy digestive systems have several things in common. Their digestive systems have always been kept highly activated as a result of digesting a lot of nutrient-dense foods. Their digestive systems don't receive undue amounts of toxic substances or food to digest on an irregular basis or during tense, stressful times. Maintaining a viable, healthy digestive system will always allow the body to efficiently digest and absorb the food it needs. Changes do occur in the digestive system, but they can be minimized.

What specific changes occur?

Years of eating will slowly grind away the teeth, although it would take 150 years or more for that to make a significant difference to anyone. The problem with teeth isn't that they wear out, but that they are lost. We are told that by the time a person reaches the age of 70, he will have lost about a third of his teeth. Maybe that's the way it has happened in the past, but it doesn't have to happen and very likely won't because of better diets, fluoridated water, and better dental care.

Another change which occurs in the mouth is the loss of taste buds. There are tiny elevations on the tongue called papillae, each one of which has 200 to 250 taste buds. By the time an individual reaches the age of 70, each papilla has less than half that amount. Whether that's a physiological loss due to aging, or a loss due to the type of food that the "average" American eats, has not yet been determined. Also, with age, the mucus membranes of the mouth secrete less fluid, making the mouth drier.

What can be done to keep the digestive system young?

If a person had to eat extra amounts of nutritious foods over a long period of time as a result of a heightened level of physical activity, it would prolong the viability of both the taste buds and the mucus membranes.

It would also enhance the muscular movement (motility) of the digestive system. Muscles of the digestive system are just like any other muscles in the body. If they are regularly exercised, they maintain their ability to contract and maintain their strength of contraction for longer periods of time. The digestive system can last well over 100 years. That is evidenced by the thousands of people who reach and pass that age. Ideally, of course, it would not only last that long, but would remain in a highly active, youthful condition.

Another thing that can be done to prolong the youthfulness of the digestive system is to avoid the ingestion of toxic substances. Trihalomethane from improperly purified water, lead from old water pipes, heavy metals such as cadmium and mercury from contaminated foods and alcohol, when consumed in excessive amounts, are all examples of toxic substances. Also, certain foods, while not toxic in moderate amounts, might have the same effect on the digestive system as do toxic substances, if consumed in excess. An intake of 40 to 50 percent of a person's calories from fat, for example, could help to prematurely age the digestive system. A lifetime of chronic overeating would also probably have this effect.

What happens to the pancreas with age?

The accessory organs of digestion also change with age. One such organ is the pancreas. The pancreas produces about a quart of pancreatic fluid each day. The fluid enters the digestive system at the small intestine's upper end near the stomach. Pancreatic fluid is primarily water, but it also contains bicarbonate to neutralize the acid from the stomach and enzymes to continue the digestive process begun there.

Enzymes in the pancreatic fluid digest carbohydrates, fats, and protein. When a balanced diet is eaten over the years—a diet containing the optimum ratio of carbohydrates, fats, and protein—the pancreas can become accustomed to producing the proper ratio of the different digestive enzymes. This will allow it to function more efficiently. On the other hand, if a diet consists of calories mostly from fat one day, mostly from protein another day, and mostly from carbohydrates on still another, the pancreas must continually adjust the ratio of the digestive enzymes that it secretes. This might cause it to function less efficiently and to deteriorate more rapidly with age.

In addition to secreting enzymes for digestion into the small intestine, the pancreas secretes insulin and other hormones directly into the bloodstream. A diet with the proper balance of carbohydrates, fats, and protein eaten at regular intervals will help keep the blood glucose level constant. The pancreas can then secrete insulin at a reasonably steady rate throughout the day. On the other hand, the ingestion of large quantities of a particular food such as sugar, at irregular intervals during the day, will cause the pancreas periodically to secrete large amounts of insulin in an attempt to control the bouncing blood glucose levels.

Poor diets aren't the only thing that have an adverse effect on the pancreas; inflammation and other conditions may affect it. Obesity, in particular, seems to overwork the pancreas and make it old before its time.

What role does the liver play in digestion?

The liver is another accessory organ of digestion. A person might be able to live without an appendix, tonsils, spleen, or other organs of the body, but he cannot live without a liver. The liver performs a myriad of functions. It collects nutrients which are absorbed from the intestine; it can transform glycogen, fat, or protein into that essential energy molecule, glycogen; it can convert any excess foods which are absorbed from the intestine into glycogen or fat, both of which can be stored in the body; and it can store minerals such as iron and copper as well as the fat-soluble vitamins—vitamins A, D, E, and K—and vitamin B12. (Some of the liver cells might be damaged if they have to store excessive amounts of vitamins.)

The liver cells break down some poisons and transform them into less harmful compounds which can be excreted. When protein is metabolized, for example, the toxic waste, ammonia, is formed. It is converted to urea by the liver, and the urea is excreted by the kidneys. Poisons which cannot be broken down and excreted remain stored in the liver.

The liver manufactures substances which can cause blood coagulation. As we go about our day-to-day activities, we cause tiny capillaries to rupture if we bump something with our hands, feet, or body. Bleeding into the tissue spaces does not occur when these tiny vessels are ruptured because the clot-forming materials produced by the liver prevent it.

The liver also produces bile salts which are transported to the small intestine to emulsify fats so that they can be more easily absorbed and digested.

What destroys liver cells and can they be regenerated?

Liver tissue is usually destroyed either by disease processes or by poisons. Many of the disease processes can be avoided, and effective treatment can be obtained for the ones which do occur. That makes it very important to give serious attention to the potential threat of poisons which can destroy liver cells. Many different poisons can injure the liver, some entering the body because of environmental pollution, others being self-administered, as in the case of chronic alcoholism.

Liver cells can regenerate; if some liver cells are destroyed, new ones will be produced until all of the destroyed ones have been replaced. That is, regeneration will occur if the blood supply remains constant, if the cells aren't destroyed too fast, and if the connective tissue which holds the cells in place remains intact.

What specific steps can I take to prevent the premature aging of my digestive system?

1. *Eat a variety of foods*, and try to keep the ratio of carbohydrates, fats, and proteins constant.

2. *Exercise daily* to increase caloric intake so that the digestive system will process a lot of food. Be sure the increased caloric intake consists of nutrient-dense foods.

3. *Drink plenty of water.* The extra fluid makes it easier for the digestive system to propel its contents along the digestive tract. Water is absorbed throughout the intestinal tract. The colon (large intestine) will absorb the necessary amount of the remaining water.

4. *Eat papaya, plums, grapes, or other fruit that supply water, fiber, and vitamin C.*

5. *Eat apples or other fiber-containing foods.* It is not necessary to load up; approximately 35 grams of fiber a day is sufficient.

6. *Occasionally eat some lean meat, yogurt, or other dairy product that contains vitamin B12.*

7. *Lay off the greasy foods.*

8. *Avoid fad diets.* Fad diets are unhealthy. In the long run they will make us fat.

9. *Avoid ingesting toxic substances* (including large amounts of fat and excess alcohol).

10. *Form good eating habits.* Insofar as possible, eat at approximately the same time each day, in quiet surroundings.

Is there a way to keep the skeletal system looking younger?

Yes, with good posture. Slouching is one sure way for a person to look older than his or her chronological age. A protruding abdomen, a rounded back, and a chin that droops weakly downward can go a long way toward helping a person take on that "I'm getting old" look. Poor posture makes a person look fatigued, and, in women, it makes the breasts appear to droop whether they do or not.

Good posture will have the reverse effect. But in order for a person to have that good posture, the skeletal system must be healthy and strong.

The bones of the body are dynamic, living structures. They offer support and protection. When the muscles contract, the bones act as levers to produce movement. The bones also serve as a depot for minerals, primarily calcium and phosphorus. The red marrow of the bones produces blood cells.

Bone continually replaces itself throughout life, allowing worn or injured bone to be removed and replaced. The replacement occurs at different rates in different areas. Since bone can be removed and replaced, and since bone is primarily calcium, it can function as a storage area for this mineral.

Why do my bones need to store calcium?

Several tissues of the body need calcium. The muscles can't contract properly without it; the nerve cells need it in order to transmit impulses; the blood cannot clot without it. The amount of calcium in the blood is very accurately controlled so that the tissues which need calcium can have it immediately. Calcium is continually being exchanged between the blood and the bones. It is removed from the bones when other tissues are not receiving enough and resupplied to the bone whenever extra calcium is available. The resupply process keeps the bones from losing bone mass.

Two things happen to the "average" person as he/she gets older. Calcium is gradually lost from the bones, and the bones become more brittle. Calcium loss begins after the age of 40 in females and after the age of 60 in males. During the next 30 years or so, the "average" female may lose as much as 30 percent of the calcium from her bones. (The joints of the "average" person also stiffen, and movement is restricted because the ligaments around the joints harden with age.)

Are my bones alive?

Indeed they are. Bones are not just solid calcium compounds; they contain protein material that allows them some degree of flexibility. In some individuals there is a decrease in the rate of formation of the protein material with age, resulting in a smaller amount of the organic protein and a greater proportion of the inorganic calcium compounds. This causes the bones to become more brittle and more susceptible to fracture.

Should I take hormones to help my bones?

I cannot answer with a simple yes or no. But let me share the result of some studies that have been done in this area. Estrogen replacement therapy has been used since the 1940s to control bone loss in post-menopausal women. The treatment became controversial when some scientific studies indicated that the hormone was linked to endometrial cancer. Later studies suggested that increased calcium in the diet could offset bone loss in post-menopausal women.

These later studies led to advertisements which claimed that everything from soup to cereal was "fortified" with calcium. Many women attempted to get the extra calcium from fancy bone meal supplements, some of which turned out to contain lead. A number of physicians, once they determine that their patients require extra calcium, prescribe two calcium-containing antacid tablets daily.

The results of yet another study have indicated that calcium supplements alone are not an adequate treatment for bone loss in post-menopausal women (*New England Journal of Medicine* 316:173-177, 1987). Three groups of early post-menopausal women were studied. One group received estrogen, a second group received oral calcium, and a third group received a placebo. The group which received estrogen therapy showed no change in bone mineral content. The group receiving the supplemental calcium and the placebo group showed a loss of bone mineral, with the loss being greater in the placebo group. The authors concluded that calcium supplements reduce bone loss, but that estrogen replacement therapy is also necessary to prevent total bone loss. But because estrogen has been linked to endometrial cancer, scientists continue to seek other ways to prevent the bone loss which accompanies aging.

What else can I do to keep my bones strong and healthy?

Aerobic exercise might be one method of preventing such loss. A study has been done on the effects of aerobic exercise on bone mass in three groups of post-menopausal women (*British Journal of Medicine* 295:1441-1444, 1987). One group regularly performed aerobic exercise for a period of one year while a second group performed the same aerobic exercises for the same period of time and also did muscle-strengthening exercises. A third group, the control group, merely continued their ordinary activities. After one year, both exercising groups had *significantly higher* bone mass than the control group. The supplemental muscle-strengthening exercises showed no additive effect on bone mass, but that aspect of the study is still under investigation. Another significant feature of the study was that the higher bone density in the exercising groups was in the trunk and upper thigh, areas which are at high risk for fractures when osteoporosis develops.

Need more be said about what prevents premature aging of the skeletal system?

CHAPTER 15

The Viability of Other Body Systems

Healthy reproductive, urinary and endocrine systems can all be carried well into old age. Many changes that we associate with aging are really a result of psychological expectations, as shown in the following story.

The late Dr. Hugh C. Keegan was an expert on venomous bites. During his career as a scientist, he often spent time in some remote corners of the world. In later years he regaled his younger colleagues with stories of his adventures. He related the following story to me at lunch one day.

While spending a few months at a remote outpost, he was approached by the mayor of the nearby village who, with a small group of men, had walked up the dirt road to the research station to speak to the scientists. The mayor had a surprising request. He had somehow gotten the mistaken idea that Dr. Keegan and his team were doing research on aphrodisiacs. He had come to them for a dose of their "miracle drug." He had to have it, as he was getting on in years, and he was scheduled to marry one of the young village maidens.

The scientists made futile attempts to explain to him the true nature of their research. He became more and more adamant about obtaining some of the miracle drug. His insistence began to border on frank hostility. Because the investigators needed the friendship of the mayor and of the people in the village, Dr. Keegan exercised the only option which seemed available to him at the time.

He disappeared into the lab and emerged with an unlabeled vial of a clear liquid—saline, a weak salt solution commonly used for intravenous fluid therapy. Dr. Keegan picked up a syringe, attached a 2-inch, 20-gauge needle to it (no pain, no gain), and drew up some of the saline. With the accuracy of a trained marksman, he bombed the bun of the venerable head of the village. The mayor's elation at getting the "miracle drug" served to offset, to some extent, the pain of the injection. He limped away back down the dirt road, massaging his hip and talking to the small entourage of lesser officials who had accompanied him on his quest. He and the young maiden were married the next day.

The scientists gave no further thought to the incident. A week later they had an anxious moment when they looked up to see the mayor again walking at a brisk pace up the dirt road toward their research station. They need not have worried. The leader was ecstatic that the miracle drug had been so effective. He made promises of enduring, lifelong friendships with everyone at the research station. He was so pleased with the wondrous power of the new drug that he wanted to return for weekly injections.

Dr. Keegan pondered the request for a moment. He then assured the mayor that the drug was so powerful that it could not be given more than once a year, that it would remain totally effective for that time, and that to give it any more often might cause adverse reactions. The village leader couldn't believe his good fortune. He could have the wonderful beneficial effect of the drug for an entire year without enduring the pain of a 20-gauge needle piercing his posterior on a weekly basis. Dr. Keegan couldn't believe his good fortune either. He knew that the mayor was happy, and he knew that he and his research team would be transferred to a new location within two months.

The above is a perfect example of why aphrodisiacs work and why some individuals remain sexually active after they are "old." They remain sexually active *because they believe they can.* The ability of individuals to remain sexually active seems more related to their general physical and mental health than to their age. Some changes do occur, such as a decrease in fertility in both males and females and a decrease in the production of the hormones estrogen and progesterone in the female, and of testosterone in the male. But these decreases in hormonal production don't preclude sexual activity.

Are there any aphrodsiacs that really work?

Not really. Powdered rhino horn, ginseng root, monkey gland transplants, oysters, and various tonics, potions, and elixirs have all been promoted as aphrodisiacs, and the search is continual. As it turns out, there is such a thing as a sexual potency diet, though it doesn't consist of exotic substances. The same foods that make the cardiovascular system healthy and the body lean, active, and energetic also promote a longer, more active sex life. Staying energetic is important. Chronic fatigue may be one of the major sexual problems in both men and women, but as we have seen, there are effective ways, including a good diet, of dealing with this condition (see Chapter Two).

What causes impotency? Is it physical or mental?

There are some physical causes of impotency, such as atherosclerosis of the vessels which supply blood to the sex organs. These organs, like all of the other organs of the body, require a good supply of blood. Thus, the same risk factors for cardiovascular disease—high blood pressure, high blood cholesterol, smoking, poor diet, and inactivity—are also risk factors for impotence caused by hardening of the arteries.

If a person is healthy, successful performance of the sexual act depends on both psychic and local stimulation. Psychic stimuli, such as simply thinking sexual thoughts, can greatly enhance a person's sexual ability. Tactile sensations are also important. Local, or tactile, sensations pass through the nerves in the pelvic region (the sacral plexus) into the lower portion of the spinal cord. From there they go up the spinal cord to the cerebrum, or the thinking part of the brain. These impulses, generated by touch, serve to reinforce the already-present psychic stimulation. When local stimulation is enhanced by appropriate conditioning impulses, or psychic stimulation, total sexual stimulation will reach maximum intensity.

The importance of psychic stimulation cannot be over-emphasized. If a growing child is taught that sex is something to be hidden, or that it is immoral, much of the natural sex drive will be inhibited. On the other hand, if a person thinks that he or she has received an aphrodisiac, as did the village mayor described above, the natural sex drive will be enhanced. These situations demonstrate the important effects that particular *beliefs* have on sexual function.

An unfortunate idea some people have is that sexual activity really isn't necessary past the age of 70, or some other arbitrary age, or that people past that age aren't "supposed" to be concerned about being sexually active. To that I say, "Balderdash." Being sexually active is much too important a part of life to be left only to the young.

Maybe some people really don't feel that it is worth changing their lifestyle in order to live to the end of their 110-year life span. I wonder if those same people would be willing to change their lifestyle in order to prevent premature impotency?

What can be done to prolong reproductive/sexual function?

1. First, and foremost, remember that *the ability to remain sexually active seems more related to general physical and mental health than to age.*

2. *Work toward maintaining general vitality with both aerobic exercise and nutrient-dense foods.*

3. *Avoid chronic fatitgue.*

4. *Don't depend too heavily on supplements* to maintain the vitality of the reproductive system. Some people claim that vitamin E (or selenium, or some other substance) helps them maintain a high level of sexual activity. (But so can an injection of an ordinary salt solution with a 20-gauge needle, if one believes in it.)

5. *Maintain the proper psychological attitude.* Don't buy the idea that sexual activity isn't important beyond a certain age, or forget that sexual interest and activity are "supposed" to decline at some point.

What is the role of the urinary system?

A noted renal physiologist, Homer Smith, once said, "The composition of the blood (and internal environment) is determined not by what the mouth ingests, but by what the kidney keeps." (Smith, H.W.: *Lectures on the Kidney*, Lawrence, Kansas, 1943, University of Kansas, page 3.) The kidneys keep some things and excrete others. By so doing, they regulate the amount of fluid in the body, the blood volume, and the blood pressure. They regulate the amount of sodium, potassium, and chlorine that is in the blood. If the kidneys fail, none of these things can be regulated; urea and other waste products cannot be eliminated from the body. In short, kidney failure, unless it is reversed or relieved by dialysis, means inevitable death.

The kidneys filter some 40 to 50 *gallons* of fluid per day, reabsorbing all of it except for approximately one quart. The kidneys normally re-absorb all of the glucose that they filter as well as varying amounts of sodium, potassium, chlorine, and other substances, depending upon the needs of the body.

Do I have any kidney filtering units to spare?

There are approximately one million filtering units called *nephrons* in each kidney. We are told that by the time an individual reaches the age of 70, he has lost approximately one-half of his nephrons. The disappearance of that number of filtering units ordinarily doesn't pose a problem, because it is possible to lead a perfectly normal life as long as approximately one-third of the nephrons remain functional (Douglas, B.H., et al, *American Journal of Physiology,* 207:669-671, 1964).

Nephrons don't just "disappear" with time. They are rendered nonfunctional by disease or injury. I once read that a scientist estimated that every time a person had one alcoholic drink he destroyed one nephron. I have no idea how he ever arrived at that particular number, but one of my colleagues remarked, "Good. That means I'll be able to have 50 drinks a day for the next 54 years, and still have half of my nephrons." Chemicals—alcohol included—do destroy nephrons, but so do other things. The point is that individuals don't *have* to lose half of their nephrons by the time they reach the age of 70.

There is a small artery which supplies blood to each of the nephrons called the afferent arteriole. If the atherosclerotic process closes that small artery, the nephron which it supplies can't function, although the nephron might have been perfectly healthy before the vessel closed. Thus, blood vessel disease can cause additional numbers of nephrons to be lost from the kidneys.

Other processes also destroy nephrons. The kidneys excrete toxins (from bacteria, for example) that can injure the nephrons. When protein is metabolized by the body, substances called nitrogenous wastes are formed. If the nephrons are required to excrete excessive amounts of these nitrogenous wastes for a prolonged period of time, their function can be affected. Certain disease processes, such as an inflammation of the kidneys (pyelonephritis), or gout, can destroy nephrons. (Gout causes uric acid to accumulate and solidify into crystals in the kidney.)

To say that the kidneys of a 70-year-old can filter waste out of the blood only half as fast as the kidneys of a 30-year-old is merely to state what happens to the average person. Since nephrons don't just disappear, an individual doesn't *have to* lose half of them by the time he reaches 70.

How can I keep my urinary system from aging prematurely?

We can do several things to prevent the premature aging of the urinary system. We can begin by *drinking adequate quantities of unpolluted water*. It isn't necessary to drink distilled water (or even water which doesn't contain minerals) as long as the water is free of pollutants. If we drink more water than we need, our kidneys will eliminate it. That might serve to "exercise" a few nephrons which otherwise would not be used.

We can *eat moderate amounts of protein*, whether the protein comes from animal or vegetable sources. If proteins supply only 15 to 20 percent of the total calories, the kidneys won't be faced with excreting large amounts of nitrogenous waste for prolonged periods of time. A lifetime of excreting wastes of this type places undue stress on the nephrons.

Many of the risk factors for heart disease are also risk factors for kidney disease. When we *adopt a lifestyle which promotes disease-free arteries*, the nephrons in our kidneys are more likely always to have an adequate blood supply. If atherosclerosis develops, the blood flow to the nephrons will be compromised.

We can, insofar as possible, *avoid the ingestion of harmful chemicals*, including excess alcohol, and heavy metals such as lead and mercury. That will help to cut our nephron losses.

Sooner or later, kidney and urinary tract problems are likely to occur in many people. *Immediate attention* to them will help preserve nephrons. Nature has provided us with approximately three times the number of nephrons that we require in order to live. People who live past the age of 100 obviously have enough nephrons to sustain life, since it is not possible to live without kidneys.

However, the more nephrons we have, the better able our kidneys are to purify our blood by filtration, to regulate blood pressure and blood volume, and to perform other vital functions.

Do our bodies have internal stabilizers?

Yes, and the stability of the internal environment of the body, homeostasis, is essential to health and vitality. Two great control systems of the body help to maintain this stability. The nervous system, discussed in another section of this book, helps maintain homeostasis by sending impulses over the neurons to all parts of the body. The nervous system can cause muscles to contract, vessels to dilate or constrict, and glands to secrete. The other control system which helps maintain homeostasis is the endocrine system.

What is the role of the endocrine system?

The endocrine system helps control the internal environment by releasing chemical messengers called hormones. It can also increase or decrease the metabolic activity of the various tissues of the body. The nervous system and the endocrine system together are sometimes referred to as the neuroendocrine system. This system regulates growth and development, ensures the survival of the individual, and enhances the survival of the species.

The endocrine system helps the body cope with emotional stress as well as with physical stresses such as pain and temperature extremes. It helps the body to adapt to, and survive, situations such as dehydration, starvation, or blood loss. The efficient functioning of the endocrine system is essential when the body is required to recover from a trauma. The endocrine system regulates the growth and development of the individual, as well as the process of reproduction. We can see that the endocrine system helps control the entire life process.

What does the pituitary gland do?

The pituitary gland is an endocrine gland embedded in the bone of the skull just beneath the brain and attached to that part of the brain known as the hypothalamus. The pituitary gland secretes hormones which influence a wide variety of body functions and hormones which stimulate other endocrine glands in the body to release their hormones. Consequently, it is sometimes referred to as the master gland.

The pituitary gland can, for example, secrete a hormone which, in turn, stimulates the adrenal glands of the body to release their hormones. (One adrenal gland sits on top of each kidney.) Hormones from the adrenal glands can raise the levels of salt and water in the blood and can help the body resist stress and inflammation.

The master gland also secretes a hormone which promotes the growth of muscle and bone. It can stimulate the thyroid gland to release hormones such as thyroxine, which helps regulate metabolism and growth. (The thyroid gland, located in the front of the neck just above its base, can also secrete calcitonin, a hormone which lowers the blood level of calcium.)

The pituitary gland secretes hormones which regulate reproduction, a hormone which can cause uterine contractions during labor, and a hormone which can cause the kidneys to conserve water. Some who study aging believe that the pituitary gland exerts an influence on the rate at which we age. That will be discussed in the next chapter.

Are there hormones that affect reproduction in the male?

Two hormones that the pituitary gland secretes affect the male reproductive system. Follicle-stimulating hormone, or FSH, stimulates the testes to produce sperm. Interstitial cell-stimulating hormone, or ICSH, stimulates the cells in the testes to produce the hormone testosterone. Testosterone promotes ''maleness,'' the development and maintenance of male secondary sex characteristics. Testosterone influences metabolism. It is known as an anabolic hormone because of its stimulating effect on protein anabolism, or growth. The body continues to produce these hormones in old age. The number of sperm cells is reduced, although abundant sperm cells may be found even in older men. This means that the pituitary gland continues to produce FSH and ICSH. Although individuals may remain sexually active as they grow older, the frequency of orgasms may be less than in young adulthood.

How do hormones affect reproduction in the female?

The pituitary gland of the female secretes several hormones which are essential to the proper functioning of the reproductive system. Two hormones, follicle-stimulating hormone, or FSH, and luteinizing hormone, or LH, stimulate the development of the ovum, or egg, the secretion of estrogens and progesterone, and ovulation.

During the female reproductive years, the blood levels of both estrogen and progesterone are higher during some days of the month than others. The changes in the blood level of these hormones is responsible for the menstrual cycle. These monthly cycles occur for a period of approximately 30 years and are manifestations of the changes in the body necessary for successful reproduction.

The cessation of the monthly menstrual cycle (menopause) does not bring a halt to sexual activity. In fact, removing the anxiety of impending pregnancy reportedly enhances sexual activity for some. Removing the uterus (hysterectomy) does not affect sexual activity either; it might also enhance sexual activity by removing the anxiety of pregnancy. The uterus is the organ that holds the fetus during development and is not an erotic organ.

What does aging do to the endocrine system?

Aging results in a reduction in the amount of some of the hormones which are produced by the endocrine system. Ordinarily this doesn't cause problems. Disorders of the endocrine system, as well as most of the difficulties which individuals encounter with respect to the endocrine system, are usually related to pathological conditions rather than age. It is essential that the endocrine system remain functional if the life span is to increase. As a matter of fact, many investigators believe that a complete understanding of the endocrine system will reveal the *key* to the aging process.

The *inappropriate* secretion of hormones from the various endocrine glands can likely contribute to premature aging as much as any other single factor. It is well known that the outpouring of hormones will age species other than humans. After salmon swim and jump their way upstream, they spawn. Then there is an outpouring of hormones from their adrenal glands. The massive amounts of the corticoid hormones poured into their bloodstreams cause them to grow old rapidly.

How does stress cause premature aging?

When humans find themselves in stressful situations for a prolonged period of time, there is an inappropriate secretion of hormones. It isn't so much that the outpouring of one particular hormone causes premature aging; it is an outpouring of several hormones *plus* a slowly developing hormonal *imbalance* that produces the premature aging.

When a person is subjected to mental and physical stress, adrenalin pours into the bloodstream. The blood pressure rises, the heart rate increases, and the person experiences the "fight or flight" reaction. Mental and physical stress stimulate the hypothalamus. Through a series of steps, other hormones are released which decrease the number of certain types of white blood cells, resulting in a decrease in the immune and allergic responses. These hormones cause a breakdown of complex, stored sugars, which elevates the blood sugar level, and increases the breakdown of tissue protein. All of these changes compromise the ability of the body to fight diseases, allergies, and infections.

Is all stress harmful?

No, if the human body is subjected to stress and then allowed a period of *recovery*, the body will be strengthened. We call this process adaptation. Problems arise when stress is so severe and so prolonged that there is permanent damage to some of the endocrine glands. When that happens, some of the endocrine glands, such as the adrenal glands, will hypertrophy (get larger). The lymphatic organs—thymus gland, spleen, and lymph nodes—will shrink. Excessive stress will produce the same changes regardless of whether the stressor is physical, as in the case of temperature extremes or exhaustion, or mental, such as worry, fear, or anxiety.

I was formerly associated with a medical center faculty member who took a bold step to eliminate a significant amount of the stress to which her body was subjected. She had morbid obesity. She had the patience and persistence to control, and eventually completely eliminate, this condition. As she lost the weight, she took up aerobic exercise—walking at first, then jogging. She eventually ran a marathon. She has significantly inhibited the premature aging of her endocrine system and the other systems of her body.

What can be done to prevent premature aging of the endocrine system?

It is worth reiterating that when disorders of the endocrine system do occur, they are more often related to pathological changes than to the aging process. However, a healthy endocrine system is *essential* for the prevention of premature aging of the entire body, and there are several ways to accomplish that.

Eliminating obesity is an important step. In the next chapter we will see how reducing the body weight of experimental animals prevents premature aging of their endocrine systems as well as other body systems and increases their life spans.

Prolonged physical and mental stress should be eliminated in order to prevent premature aging of the endocrine system. A high-powered, fast-paced, exciting career and lifestyle can be wonderful and invigorating; but occasionally it is necessary to take some time to smell the roses, or to go to the seashore and build some sand castles. The recovery period will serve to strengthen the entire body.

Eat nutrient-dense foods. They will provide a person with all of the required vitamins and minerals and enhance the vitality of the endocrine system and all other systems. Collards, cold-water fish, dried beans, or other foods which contain niacin will help. Niacin deficiency depresses all of the functions of the body, causing, among other things, muscle weakness and poor glandular secretion. Cereal will provide chromium which potentiates the action of insulin. Seafoods and iodized salt will provide the iodine necessary for the formation of thyroxin.

A lifestyle that benefits the cardiovascular system will also help keep the endocrine system healthy. The endocrine glands need a good supply of oxygen-rich blood if they are going to function at peak efficiency for a prolonged period of time. *A routine of daily aerobic exercise* sends signals to the brain, the endocrine system, and all of the other systems of the body that they are to remain healthy and functional.

CHAPTER 16

Now That I'm 110 Years Old, What's Next?

We have finally freed ourselves from the cocoon of ignorance, prejudice, and superstition which made us cling for so long to the belief that we couldn't change the life span. That freedom has allowed us to enter a new era. We now know that we can exert a significant influence on the rate at which we age and essentially prevent premature aging.

Can the human life span be extended?

Yes, it can. Scientists have extended the life span of several different species of animals by 30 to 40 percent, and more. If a given stimulus produces a particular response in several different species of animals, it will almost always produce the same, or a similar response in humans. Therefore, it seems likely that stimuli that extend the life span of other species will do the same for humans. Here's why:

Muscle, kidney, and liver function, and the function of the other systems of the body, are almost identical in many different species of animals, including rodents, dogs, chimpanzees, and humans. If a hormone is released in response to a particular stimulus in chimpanzees or dogs, for example, it will likely do the same in humans. If a drug will lower blood pressure in the spontaneously hypertensive rat, it will probably do the same in humans. Fertilization, maturation, and aging all occur in a very similar fashion in those different animals. Thus, there is a high degree of probability that any process that retards aging in one species will retard aging in another.

We haven't always known how to prevent premature aging of the different systems of the body, and it has only been in very recent times that scientists have been able to extend the life span of experimental animals. Not knowing how to do these things made us believe that we couldn't do them. Now that we have gotten past that barrier, progress is being made rather rapidly. An extension of the human life span by 30 to 40 percent would mean that humans could live to be 140 to 150 years old.

How did we come to suspect that there is an aging clock in the first place?

We came to suspect that there is an aging clock because of the fact that different animal species live for different lengths of time. After animals—humans included—are born, they mature, grow old, and die. Animals don't grow old just because of the passing of time. If that were so, they would all age at the same rate and live the same length of time.

Inside all of us—inside all animals—is an aging clock that is ticking away. The reason that different animal species have different life spans is that their aging clocks are set differently. If everything works perfectly for the laboratory rat, it will live for about three years. If everything works perfectly for the human—no diseases, no accidents—the human will live for about 110 years. At the end of three years the rat will die, and at the end of 110 years the human will die *because that is the way their biological aging clocks have been programmed.* If the laboratory rat and the human are to live much beyond these life spans, their aging clocks will have to be changed.

How can life span be determined?

Determining life span is relatively easy with animals such as mice, which live only a few months. A large number of them can be placed in a controlled environment and observed to see how long they live. Determining the life span of animals who live longer is possible through the examination of records kept by zoos all over the world. Careful birth and death records are also kept for thoroughbred animals and provide information about their life spans.

Gathering data on humans is a little more difficult. Today, birth and death records are commonly kept, but that hasn't always been the case. Birth registration is a relatively recent (19th century) development. Birth records, together with an assessment of the biological markers of aging, make it possible to fairly accurately pinpoint the human life span at 110 years.

What happens if we cure all diseases and prevent all accidents?

If additional research allows us to cure all diseases and prevent all accidents, we will all live to be 110 years old. That, theoretically, will be the end of medical progress. We won't be able to live longer than 110 years by doing research on other diseases. We will be able to live longer only if we find ways to slow the aging clock.

Because we *have* found preventions and cures for diseases including some of the cancers, the human life expectancy has increased dramatically. (We're still making progress on preventing and curing diseases, including cancer. We know that diet and environment are probably responsible for 80 to 90 percent of the cancers, while only 10 to 20 percent are genetic in origin. That allows cancer researchers to know where to focus their efforts.) Life expectancy has increased, but the maximum survival time, or life span, hasn't changed, because it is determined by the biological aging clock.

Is premature aging just a fact of life?

We can take two approaches to the aging process. We can simply accept premature aging and a fixed life span as a fact of life, then wax philosophical about it and forget it, or we can do something about it. Apparently people generally don't want to go along the way they are for the rest of their lives, but are willing to see if there are better and more exciting things in store for them—to see if they can do something about slowing the aging process.

Some individuals believe that we shouldn't experiment with increasing the human life span because it's against the "natural order of things." I find that difficult to accept. To me, it's no more against the natural order of things than was cleaning up the drinking water to prevent diseases or finding a cure for diseases such as smallpox and polio.

Who wants an extended stay in the nursing home?

Extending life span doesn't mean that we are merely going to add more years in the nursing home. No one wants that. Extending the life span will allow people to be younger for a much longer period of time, to *stretch out the middle years*. We can't let our attitudes about research on life span be influenced by the mind-set of the past which decreed that one is supposed to get ''old'' at 65, spend a few years in retirement, a few years in the nursing home, and then die.

This concept of aging has caused many people to look upon old age as totally undesirable and to see no point in attempting to prolong it. If scientific investigators felt that way, it would impede progress in aging research. Fortunately, this antiquated view of aging is passing from the scene.

Can aging be slowed by restricting the diet?

Yes. That is the one *known* stimulus that will slow the aging clock: food restriction. It slows the aging of *all* of the systems of the body. In other words, *food restriction retards a basic aging process.* Since food restriction has that effect on several different species of experimental animals, it is reasonable to expect the same result in humans. (The food must be restricted in a particular fashion, as discussed below. Starvation and malnutrition don't slow the aging clock.)

In the lower animal, all of the indicators of aging which have been measured can be significantly slowed by manipulating the diet. That the diet can be manipulated to extend life span was observed years ago (McCay, 1934), but that observation lay dormant for a time. McCay conducted his experiments because he thought that all aging took place after maturity. His initial plan was to keep his experimental animals from reaching maturity by feeding them less food. Actually he wanted to keep them the size they were at birth, but he was unable to reduce their food intake that drastically and still keep them alive.

McCay was not able to keep his animals from reaching maturity, but he made another observation. *By reducing their food intake, he was able to increase their life span.* He wrongly thought that he had increased their life span because he was able to delay their maturing. In reality, it was the food restriction that extended the life span of the animals. Later studies have shown that food restriction which is started in animals after they become adults is just about as effective at increasing their life span. Later investigators (Walford, Yu, Masoro, Weindruch, Hart, and others) were able to substantially improve upon McCay's experiments by a process they refer to as *under*nutrition without *mal*nutrition. The concept is to *reduce the total caloric intake while giving the animals all of the required vitamins and minerals, plus a proper balance of carbohydrates, fats, and protein.*

The scientists found that when they fed their animals a diet with a reduced caloric intake, but *without malnutrition*, the animals fared better if the calories and the essential nutrients came from *food* instead of supplements. Animals placed on a totally synthetic diet, even though with proper amounts of all of the known essential vitamins, minerals, and other nutrients, did not fare well.

The different systems of the body age with time. The muscles, heart, lungs, kidneys, and other organs show characteristic age-related changes. Reducing the caloric intake (without malnutrition) not only increases the life span, but also inhibits the basic aging process of all of the different systems of the body. It also delays the onset and slows the development of age-related diseases. The life span, a programmed event, increases. Caloric restriction slows the aging clock.

What does caloric restriction do?

Food restriction inhibits most of the natural changes that occur as animals age. It inhibits the basic aging processes of all of the different systems of the body. It delays the onset and slows the development of age-related diseases.

The wrinkling of the skin, loss or graying of hair, and other changes which occur with time are *programmed* changes. Extending the human life span only requires that the built-in program for aging be changed. Food restriction somehow alters that program. This has been demonstrated by several investigators (Yu, Masoro, Walford, Weindruch, Hart, and others).

A typical experiment consists of raising two groups of animals such as mice (which have a short life span) in a controlled environment. One group is allowed to have as much food as they want, whenever they want it, throughout their lives. That amount of food is measured. The food intake of the second group of animals is restricted to 60 percent of the amount of food that the first group eats. Then both groups of animals are simply allowed to grow old and die. The animals on the reduced food intake typically live 35 to 50 percent longer, and usually about 75 percent of them are still alive when all of the animals on the high-food intake have died. The food restriction actually increases life span, provided that the food which the animals do receive is highly nutritious. No other form of anti-aging therapy even comes close to being as effective as food restriction in increasing the life span. This technique is effective in increasing the life span even if restriction is begun after the animals become adults.

Food restriction has several results. Connective tissue throughout the body holds all of the organs together; the main constituent of this tissue is a substance called collagen. Food restriction slows the aging of collagen.

Food restriction almost totally prevents the age-related increase in blood cholesterol. What's more, the HDL and LDL factors remain at the same favorable ratio as in younger animals. The food-restricted animals frequently have blood-cholesterol levels as low as or lower than cholesterol levels in the fully fed animals which are half their age (Masoro, *Journal of the American Geriatrics Society* 32:296, 1984).

Walford (see references) has written extensively, recipes included, about increasing the human life span by caloric restriction. If we are to translate from the animal experiments as Walford and others do, the human body weight should be reduced to approximately 10 to 20 percent below the "setpoint."

What is the setpoint?

The setpoint is probably the average weight during the young adult years, during a time when the individual was neither dieting nor overeating. This implies that all individuals would not have to strive for the same absolute body weight, but for a 10 to 20 percent reduction in setpoint.

We all have different setpoints for body weight. One person's setpoint might be at a normal weight (according to standard height-weight charts), another's at a weight that would make him slightly obese, and still another's at a level that would make him very obese.

If a person with a normal body weight reduces his setpoint for body weight by 10 to 20 percent, his weight will be below the weight level of the standard height-weight charts. If an obese person reduces his setpoint for body weight by 10 to 20 percent, he might then have a normal weight. Yet when the obese person reduces his weight by that amount, he will increase his life expectancy and possibly his life span. Scientific studies bear this out. When genetically obese rats are calorie restricted so that they have a normal body weight, their life span increases.

If we were to undertake a 10 to 20 percent reduction in body weight setpoint in order to increase our life span, it would still be necessary to get *all* of the essential nutrients that our bodies require. Caloric restriction alone is not sufficient. Malnutrition (even with an adequate supply of calories) and starvation both *decrease* the life span. Also, if we are to translate from Walford's animal experiments, these weight reductions should occur over a four-to-six-year period. When the weight reduction occurs slowly, the metabolic efficiency increases. Extra calories aren't burned without benefit. Excess metabolic end-products aren't formed for the body to have to eliminate.

Who wants to live more than 110 years, anyway?

This is a question that people must answer for themselves. If extending the life span means stretching out the middle years of life—extending the number of "young" years—it is well worth considering. Experiments have not been done in humans, as they have in experimental animals, to demonstrate that dietary manipulation will increase the life span, but we don't have time to wait around to see how lifetime experiments in humans will work out.

If such experiments were conducted and proved fruitful, that would be good news for future generations, although it would do little good for those of us who are now alive.

What if you tried extending your life span by caloric restriction and it didn't work?

It would probably still increase your life expectancy by reducing the early incidence of degenerative diseases. It would probably add on 10 or more "young" years.

How do our genes affect the aging clock?

The rate at which the aging clock ticks in any species is determined ultimately by the genetic make-up of that species. Humans have a multitude of genes in their cells. The genetic program for aging is probably "written" (contained) in only a few of the genes; it almost certainly doesn't involve all of the hereditary material in the cells of the body.

Various tissues of the body are composed of different types of cells. Muscle cells, liver cells, and kidney cells, though not alike, all contain the same genes. Only certain genes function in each cell type, depending upon what the cell is required to do. The genes that are functional in the muscle cells are not the same genes that are functional in the liver cells and vice versa. The genes that are not functional are said to be "repressed;" those that are operating are said to be "expressed." The nature of gene expression is not clearly understood. It is not known why certain genes are functional in muscle cells and others are functional in liver cells. As that comes to be understood, as it eventually will, the cellular clock might be understood and manipulated. If aging is a part of gene expression, it might be possible to manipulate the genes into not "turning on" the aging process.

There are other theories regarding the mechanism of aging. Some scientists believe that the initiating event in aging is the appearance of a destructive agent. That would seem to assume that aging begins after maturity, a theory postulated by McCay in 1934. Destructive agents do appear and cause aging in one or two species. Walford (1986) mentioned the octopus as an example. Aging is caused by a massive hormone release in the octopus, and if the gland which releases the hormone is removed, the octopus lives up to five times its normal life span. The identification of such a substance in the human (if it does exist) would be logically followed by attempts to neutralize and/or inhibit the release of the substance.

Another phenomenon which has attracted the attention of scientists who are interested in the aging process is that the life spans of various species of animals seem to be proportional to their ability to repair their DNA.

How important is the ability to repair DNA?

Animals that repair it quickly have a longer life span. Apparently certain enzymes in the body identify the injury to DNA, and the injury is then repaired. The mouse, whose life span is a few months, repairs DNA slowly, while the human, whose life span is 110 years, repairs DNA rapidly. (DNA is damaged as a result of normal metabolism and harmful agents entering the body.)

The rate of DNA repair might well be a factor responsible for aging since humans with the disease known as Down's syndrome show defects in the DNA repair system, and Down's syndrome causes premature aging. The possibility exists that the human body can be stimulated to increase its level of repair enzymes. It seems likely that we will learn how to increase the level of the repair process of DNA within the cells of the human body, since it has already been done in the one-cell animal.

What about the theory of energy consumption?

Almost every time I talk to a group of people about the mechanisms of aging, someone mentions the theory of energy consumption. This is an idea which has been bandied about from time to time. Almost all animals use approximately the same number of calories—25 to 40 million—per pound per lifetime. Humans are the exception to the general rule. They consume approximately 80 million calories per pound in a lifetime. These facts have prompted some scientists to propose that each animal has a fixed amount of energy that it can use in its lifetime. Once the allotted number of calories has been used, the life span will be at an end. Some groups of people burn many more calories on a daily basis than others. Yet, the life span of all humans is about the same. There is a considerable variation in the life span of the different species of animals, and the number of calories that they burn per pound in a lifetime might be coincidence rather than cause and effect.

Can cell division be turned on and off?

Indications are that it can. In the 1960s Dr. Leonary Hayflick made an interesting observation about human fibroblasts. (As you may recall, fibroblasts are cells that are found in the connective tissue of the body.) Dr. Hayflick observed that human fibroblasts, when grown in culture, won't divide more than about 50 times. As the 50th division approaches, the cells begin to divide more slowly, and microscopic examination of them reveals age-related changes. Finally the cells don't divide at all. Fibroblasts from young people undergo more divisions than those from older people. This "Hayflick number," indicates that aging is an intrinsic part of the cellular process; that there is a biological clock ticking away within each cell. At least that's the way it works in fibroblasts. Fifty doublings of the fibroblasts are called the "Hayflick limit." Some who study aging have proposed that all of the cells of the body go through a given number of divisions, and when the divisions are complete, the life span is over. Whether all varieties of cells conform to the Hayflick limit is not known. Cancer cells certainly don't; they'll divide forever, as long as they are fed. This indicates that cell division can be turned on and off, and that there is an overall regulator.

What about the immune theory of aging?

Some scientists believe that changes in the immune system are responsible for the aging process. The immune system recognizes "self" and "nonself," seeking out and destroying anything that is nonself. Unfortunately, as people grow older, the surface of the body cells changes. Because of this and/or because the immune system doesn't function as efficiently with the passing of time, the immune system sometimes turns on "self." According to the immune theory of aging, the more the surface of the cells of the body changes, the more likely the immune system is to form antibodies to attack the body's own cells. This may be a partial explanation, but we have to wonder why the cell surfaces change faster in some animals than in others. We have to wonder why the immune system turns against its own cells faster in the mouse than it does in the human. It seems reasonable to propose that there is an overall "controller" of life span which orchestrates these changes at different rates in the different species.

What could this overall controller of life span be?

The hypothalamus might be the controller. At a certain time in life, the hypothalamus programs hormonal variations and has the pituitary gland elaborate certain hormones to bring on puberty. The aging clock itself might well be in the hypothalamus. It could program hormonal variations to be carried out by the pituitary gland to regulate the onset and the rate of aging. The aging clock in the hypothalamus could then have the immune system and the entire neuroendocrine system serve as the pacemakers of the aging process.

Whatever the nature of the aging clock, we do know that it can be slowed in a number of different species and that there is a high probability that it can also be slowed in humans.

Is there one single thing that has affected all our biological aging markers?

Every single biological marker for aging which has been studied is affected by caloric restriction. For example, as animals get older, the blood level of the hormone calcitonin increases. This is undesirable because it lowers the amount of calcium in the blood. Food restriction prevents these changes.

Muscle cells are lost as animals get older. (There isn't much loss of muscle cells from the diaphragm, the large muscle of respiration, probably because it is continually exercised.) In addition to the loss, degenerative changes occur in the muscle cells that remain. Food restriction delays these changes (R.J.M. Carter, et al, *American Journal of Physiology* 242:89, 1982). Food restriction also inhibits the age-related changes and loss of smooth muscle, which is found in the walls of the intestine and the ureter, in the blood vessels, and elsewhere in the body.

The fat cells in the body become less sensitive to several hormones with age. The hormone glucagon can act to raise the blood sugar level, if necessary. In fully fed rats, the response of fat cells to this hormone falls to zero by the time they are six months old. Caloric restriction prolongs this response. At the age of twelve months, the response is essentially the same as in three-month-old animals, and the food-restricted animals are able to respond to it throughout their lifetimes.

Food restriction prevents the age-related rise in blood insulin and blood sugar levels. With age, the tissues tend to become resistant to the effects of insulin, but caloric restriction prevents the development of the resistance (Reavan and Reavan, *Metabolism* 30:982, 1981).

Food restriction also prevents the age-related loss in bone mass and the loss of certain types of receptors in the brain, keeps the immune system younger for a longer period of time, and maintains the body's ability to repair its own DNA.

The development of age-related diseases such as chronic nephropathy (kidney disease) is dramatically reduced under this program. In one study (Yu, 1984) food restriction so successfully slowed the development of chronic nephropathy that almost none of the animals on the restricted diet had the disease, while 72 percent of the group on the high food intake did have it. Reduced food intake also delayed the development of cardiomyopathy, a disease of the heart muscle, and the development of lymphomas.

Then caloric restriction may be the key to slowing the aging clock?

It very well may be the single most important factor. Food restriction not only delays the rate of aging in the experimental animals, but the animals also *live younger longer*. This demonstrates the very broad way in which food restriction affects the changes that occur with age. *Everything in the body is affected because food restriction is slowing the aging clock.*

These are not the hare-brained ideas of some movie star, someone with a smattering of scientific knowledge, or some other layperson who has decided to become a "medical authority." This evidence has come from some of the most respected scientific laboratories in the world.

Extending the life span will postpone age-related as well as man-made diseases. Diseases which begin to occur at the age of 40 might not begin to occur until the age of 90. An 80-year-old whose life span has been increased might be as physiologically young as today's 60-year-olds. We will completely eliminate the false notion that people somehow aren't the same simply because they have lived a specific number of years. Chronological age will be even less an indicator of functional age than it is now. Many of the problems of old age will be eliminated because the middle years will have been increased.

A Closing Word

Legitimate scientists don't claim that they can make people live forever. They do know that it's now possible to intervene and prevent and/or inhibit many of the processes associated with aging. We will see people not only living longer, but living younger—living to the very end of the maximum life span, then dying while still physically and mentally active.

Our biological clocks are going to go right on ticking, but there are some exciting new areas of research. Genes, hormones, cellular metabolic mechanisms, and immune system boosters are all being investigated. By the time we reach the end of our 110-year life span, new drugs and treatments will be available that will make it possible for the chronologically old to be even more functionally young than they are today.

Our lives are not really influenced by the arrangement of the stars in the galaxy, or by mysterious, unseen forces. They are more likely to be influenced by the people we meet, the experiences we have, and the books we read. I hope my message will influence you to be young, and to remain young to the very end of your life span.

References

Alexander, Nancy "Fish oils inhibit autoimmune disease" *FASEB Newsletter* 20(6):6, 1987.

Berenson, G.S., et al., "Review: Atherosclerosis and its evolution in childhood" *The American Journal of the Medical Sciences* 294:429, 1987.

Butler, R.N. "Successful aging and the role of the life review" in *Aging*, (H. Cox, Ed.), p. 16, Dushkin Publishing Group, Inc. Guilford, Conn, 1985.

Chernoff, R., and Lipschitz, D. A. (editors) *Health Promotion and Disease Prevention in the Elderly*, Raven Press, Ltd., New York, N.Y., 1988

Christensen, Susan G. "Charity Begins at Home" in *The Clarion-Ledger*, (Jackson, MS), p. E-1, April 1, 1990.

Conniff, R. "Living longer" in *Aging*, (H. Cox, Ed.), p. 48, Dushkin Publishing Group, Inc. Guilford, Conn, 1985.

Cox, Harold, *Annual Editions Series: Aging* (4th Ed.), Dushkin Publishing Group, Inc., Guilford, Conn., 1985.

Douglas, Ben H., *Reset Your Appestat*, QRP Books, Brandon, MS., 1988.

Douglas, B.H., Guyton, A.C., Langston, J.B., and Bishop, V.S. "Hypertension caused by salt loading: II. Fluid volume and tissue pressure changes." *American Journal of Physiology* 207:669-671, 1964.

Dumesnil, Jean G. "Running and weightlifting build the heart" *FASEB Newsletter* 21(7):6, 1988.

Film: "How to live to be 140: Extending our Biological Limits," Catalog No. F612.67-TOL, Mississippi State University, Starkville, MS.

Food and Nutrition Board. *Recommended Dietary Allowances* (9th rev. ed.), Washington, D.C.: National Academy of Sciences, National Research Council, 1980.

Gori, G.B., *Cancer* 43:2151, 1979.

Friedman, Meyer, *Type-A Behavior and Your Heart*, Random House, New York, N.Y., 1974

Glasser, William, *Positive Addiction*, Harper & Row, New York, N.Y., 1976.

Hall, E. "Acting one's age: New rules for old" in *Aging*, (H. Cox, Ed.), p. 10, Dushkin Publishing Group, Inc. Guilford, Conn., 1985.

Herbert, Victor "Health claims in food labeling and advertising: Literal truths but false messages; deceptions by omission of adverse facts" *Nutrition Today*, P. 25, May/June 1987.

Holman, Susan R., *Essentials of Nutrition for the Health Professions*, J. B. Lippincott Company, Publishers, Philadelphia, 1987.

Kroenke, K., et. al. "Chronic fatigue in primary care. Prevalence, patient characteristics, and outcome. *Journal of the American Medical Association* 260 (7): 929-34, 1988.

Lew, E.A., and Garfinkel, L. "Variations in mortality by weight among 750,000 men and women." *Journal of Chronic Diseases* 32:563-576, 1979.

Lyte, M. and Shinitzky, *Biochemica et Biophysica Acta* 812:133, 1985.

Mann, G. V., et al. "Atherosclerosis in the Masai" *American Journal of Epidemiology* 95:26, 1972.

Mann, G.B., et al. "Physical fitness and immunity to heart disease in Masai" *Lancet* 2:1308-1310, 1965.

Masoro, E. "State of knowledge on action of food restriction on aging." *Basic Life Science* 35:105-116, 1985.

Masoro, E.J. "Aging and nutrition-can diet affect life span?" *Transactions of the Association of Life Insurance Medical Directors of America* 67:30-44, 1985.

McCay, C. M., Crowell, M.F. and Maynard, L.M. "The effect of retarded growth upon the length of life span and upon ultimate body size." *Journal of Nutrition* 10:63-70, 1935.

Michalopoulos, G.K. "Liver regeneration: molecular mechanisms of growth control" *The FASEB Journal* 4(2):176, 1990.

Nielsen, F.H. "Boron is essential" *FASEB Newsletter*, p. 6, April, 1989.

Paffenbarger, R.S., Jr., Hyde, R.T., Wing, A.L. and Hsieh, C. "Physical activity, all-cause mortality, and longevity of college alumni." *The New England Journal of Medicine* 314(10):605-613, 1986.

Pritikin, Nathan, *The Pritikin Program for Diet & Exercise*, Bantam Books, pp, 28, 69-70, New York, N.Y., 1979.

Sasaki, Jun, et al. "Mild exercise therapy increases serum high density lipopotrein cholesterol levels in patients with essential hypertension" *The American Journal of the Medical Sciences* 297(4):220, 1989.

Shekelle, R. *New England Journal of Medicine* 304:65-70, 1981.

Taylor, A. "Moderate caloric restriction delays cataract formation in the Emory mouse" *The FASEB Journal* 3:1741, 1989.

Tortora, G.J. *Principles of Human Anatomy*, Harper & Row, Publishers, New York, 1986.

Tierney, J. "The aging body" in *Aging* (H. Cox, Ed.), p. 54, Dushkin Publishing Group, Inc., Guilford, Conn., 1985.

Walford, R.L., *The 120-year diet*, Pocket Books, New York, 1986.

Weindruch, R. et al., *Age* 5:111, 1982.

Weindruch, R. and Walford, R.L., *Science* 215:1415, 1982.

Weindruch, R. et al., "The retardation of aging in mice by dietary restriction: Longevity, cancer, immunity and lifetime energy intake" *Journal of Nutrition* 116:641, 1986.

Wilkins, R.W. and Levinsky, N.G. (Eds.), *Medicine*, 3rd Edition, Little, Brown and Co., Boston, 1983.

Yu, B.P., Masoro, E.J., Murata, I. Bertrand, H.A. and Lynd, F.T. "Life span study of SPF Fisher 344 male rats fed ad libitum or restricted diets: Longevity, growth, lean body mass and disease." *Journal of Gerontology* 37:130-141, 1982.

Zeller, Kathleen R. "Review: Effects of dietary protein and phosphorus restriction on the progression of chronic renal failure" *The American Journal of the Medical Sciences* 294(5):328, 1987.

Of Related Interest

Reset Your Appestat*

by Dr. Ben H. Douglas

Reset Your Appestat is a weight control book that is not a diet book. It is a successful program fro achieving permanent weight control without rigid diets or strenuous exercise.

In this book, Dr. Douglas gives a detailed, easy-to-follow methodology for lowering the appestat, the body's built-in regulator of appetite and satiety. There are no recipes to follow, no pills to take, no equipment to order, no starvation from eating the foods you are accustommed to eating. The method requires only that you follow Dr. Douglas' guidelines for resetting your appestat by using carefully prescribed repetitive processes. The weight comes off gradually, correctly,... and stays off.

Dr. Douglas has developed and perfected a method of weight control that may become the only method people use to control their weight. It will be around for a long time because it makes sense and it works. It is already within everybody to be at his/her ideal weight—it's just a matter of regulating the appestat. You can also reset your appestat higher if you want to gain weight.

Even if your appestat is already set at the desired level, the book is full of good reading for anybody who has concern for their physical well-being.

ISBN 0-937552-21-6
208 pages, hardbound, $12.95

---

*(ăp′ e-stăt′) n. Appetite thermostat. The mechanism in the central nervous system that controls food intake.